KIMINTA

A Maasai's Fight
against Female Genital Mutilation

Memoir and Sourcebook

KIMINTA

A Maasai's Fight
against Female Genital Mutilation

Memoir and Sourcebook

Maria Kiminta and Tobe Levin
Photographs by Britta Radike

UnCUT/VOICES Press
2015

ISBN: 978-3-9813863-6-3

Bibliographic information published by the Deutsche Nationalbibliothek.
The Deutsche Nationalbibliothek lists this publication in the Deutsche
Nationalbibliografie; detailed bibliographic data are available on the internet at
http://dnd.d-nb.de
Frankfurt am Main: UnCUT/VOICES Press, 2015.

UnCUT/VOICES Press
Martin Luther Str. 35, 60389 Frankfurt am Main, Germany
Tobe.levin@uncutvoices.com www.uncutvoices.com
www.uncutvoices.wordpress.com
Geschäftsnummer HRB 86527, U.G. Haftungsbeschränkt

Also from UnCUT/VOICES PRESS

Khady with Marie-Thérèse Cuny. *Blood Stains. A Child of Africa Reclaims Her
Human Rights*. Trans. Tobe Levin. ISBN: 978-3-9813863-0-1
A ground-breaking memoir by Senegalese Khady, Europe's leading activist against
female genital mutilation, forced and early marriage, and unequal gender relations
in the African Diaspora. "Khady's account ... is wrenching and necessary reading."
- Henry Louis Gates, Jr., Harvard University

Hubert Prolongeau. *Undoing FGM. Pierre Foldes, the Surgeon Who Restores
the Clitoris*. Foreword by Bernard Kouchner, founder of Doctors without Borders
and former Foreign Minister of France. Trans. and Afterword by Tobe Levin.
ISBN: 978-3-9813863-1-8.
"Can excision be reversed? Can the wounded sex be healed? French surgeon
Pierre Foldes ... return[s] to eager patients their sensitivity, femininity, and courage
to break the chain. A must read!" – Elfriede Jelinek, 2004 Nobel Laureate in Literature

Nick Hadikwa Mwaluko. *WAAFRIKA. Kenya. 1992. Two Women Fall in Love*.
Foreword by Ginni Stern. ISBN: 978-3-9813863-2-5
"Powerful and fearless, ... Mwaluko's ground-breaking drama challenges our local
and global imaginings of African love and sexual identity." – Tracie Jones,
Harvard Graduate School of Education

Tobe Levin, ed. *Waging Empathy. Alice Walker, Possessing the Secret of Joy and
the Global Movement to Ban FGM*. ISBN: 978-3-9813863-3-2
"With enthusiasm I endorse these essays from around the world showing that
readers and critics alike appreciate a story about FGM. Our stories will end the
scourge once and for all." – Soraya Miré, filmmaker and author.

Frankie Hutton, ed. *Rose Lore. Essays in Cultural History and Semiotics*.
ISBN: 978-3-981386349.
"The archetypal rose allows us to breathe human meaning into a non-human part
of the physical world that constitutes our common heritage." -- Dr. Maria Jaschok,
International Gender Studies at Lady Margaret Hall, University of Oxford (with a
chapter by Tobe Levin on "FGM, or Cutting the Rose in Alice Walker's Garden.")

Cover acrylic: Godfrey Williams-Okorodus, *Kiminta*, 2014

TABLE OF CONTENTS

*With gratitude to the *International Journal of Innovation and Scientific Research*. This edited chapter is used here under provisions applying to an "open access article distributed under the Creative Commons Attribution License, which permits unrestricted use, distribution, and reproduction in any medium, provided the original work is properly cited." Proper citation accompanies the chapter.

This book is dedicated to proud Maasai girls –
educated, intact, and happy to enhance their own
and others' lives.

Acknowledgments

Maria Kiminta would like to express special appreciation to her pastor
Silke Häß, to the Claudia Kühlman family, to the VHS Kaltenkirchen and especially Astrid Kruse, to the church in Kaltenkirchen that supported her and,
of course, to her publisher Tobe Levin.

Tobe Levin thanks Maria Kiminta for trust and, especially, patience, during
the extended length of this project. Gratitude is also due to Dr. Maria
Jaschok and International Gender Studies at Lady Margaret Hall, University of Oxford, where, as a Visiting Research Fellow in 2014-2015, she
enjoyed the opportunity to pursue Female Genital Mutilation Studies and
bring this book to fruition.

PREFACE

Maria Kiminta

Joy sat down with me when I first conceived of writing this book. Motivated by my own need for answers, I knew that others, too, wanted broader knowledge. Like me, they would welcome the chance to move beyond the static information of the past. And even if immediate success eluded me (would I find a publisher? would my writing hit the mark?), communicating what I had learned, I was bold enough to think, could alter African culture, both in the Diaspora, – including where I live, in Germany –, and in Africa. For traditions responsible for FGM and the risk it poses to girls' health are cultural, and therefore stubborn, but culture and destiny can change. Written and spoken words, sincerity and conscientious action can realize African people's aspirations for their children.

If coming generations are to become innovative, resourceful leaders, they need role models. I dared to use my education to become such a leader, at least insofar as memoir reaches out, explaining in this text which fixed beliefs permit the use of razors against girls and why my desire to see those girls evade the blades can be realized after all.

When I was growing up in Kenya, I had a single option, to become someone's wife. It was drilled into me that we are Maasai (or, speaking for my friends, Kikuyu) and, even if we didn't brew traditional beer like other Maasai, we were still a people apart. The past remained present and the present – its encroachments – was resisted. At times, these constant comparisons to the ways of life now slowly invading our domain made us feel that we were better than, although often enough less than, those practicing another culture.

But the other culture's benefits – computers, cures for diseases, kidney transplants – have made me thankful, as an African woman, for the new technology, and gratitude trusts in change.

It is the source of my yearning to liberate children, above all, from the emotional and cultural bondage that molded us and affected our whole lives. I would say to my people, please focus on today and let go of the past. Choose to alter – culture and yourselves.

Rooted as it is in the past, FGM must end.

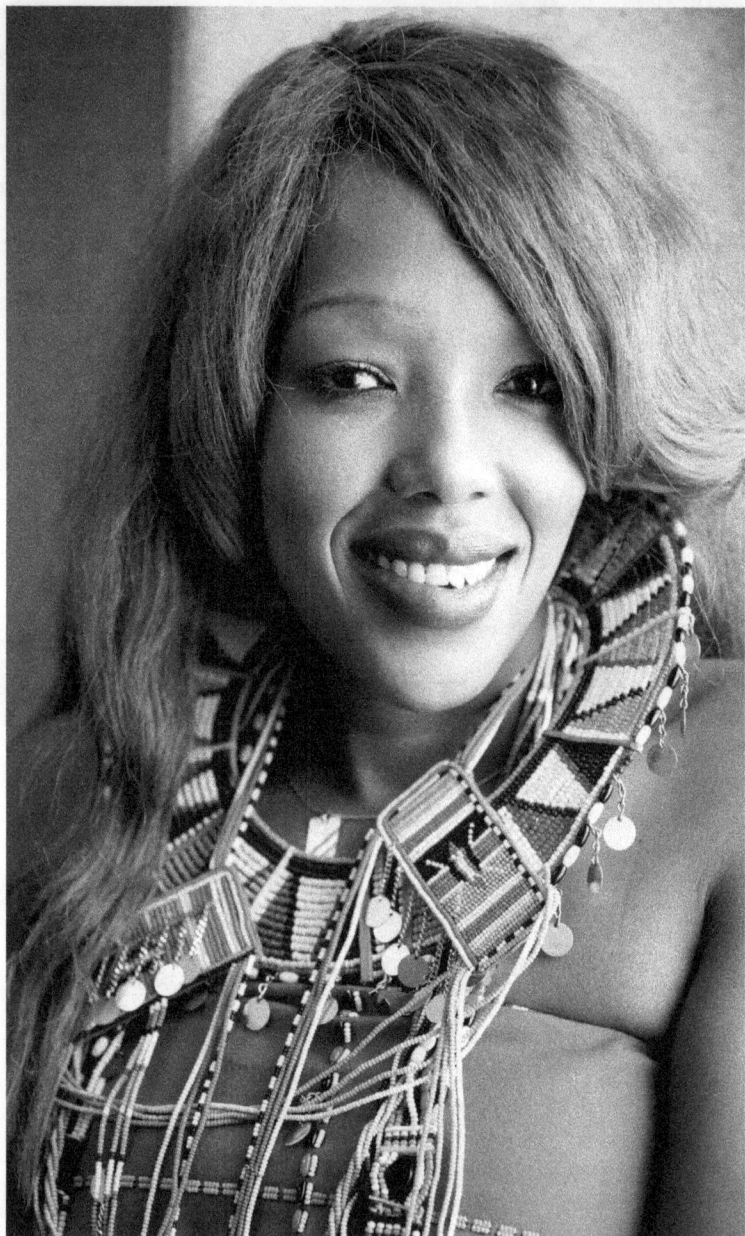

KIMINTA
A Maasai's Fight
against Female Genital Mutilation

Memoir and Sourcebook

I am a Maasai, and I was subjected to female genital mutilation.

Although commonly called "circumcision" by people not (yet) ready to abandon the practice, the rite involves slicing off parts of the visible female genitalia or otherwise injuring sex-ual organs for reasons other than malignancy, malformation or illness. Not medically prescribed, the 'surgery' answers cultural, religious or other non-therapeutic mandates. Recent reports observe a shift – minor among the Maasai – towards medicalization of the process, now increasingly offered by trained personnel ostensibly to limit side effects and pain. But in case you are tempted to smile, this is *not* a positive development and is, in fact, strongly opposed by, among others, the Inter-African Committee.[1]

A long-standing cultural practice, Female Genital Mutilation (FGM) is not limited to my community but prevails equally in other pastoral ethnic groups. Although girls between four and ten are its most frequent victims, it takes place at any age from infancy through adolescence. Although thirteen to sixteen years had been preferred where I grew up, now, to avoid detection by authorities, clitoridectomy is often performed on babies.

As children, we were meant to believe that FGM is a 'good tradition'. This would be elaborated to us by the old women and grandparents during evening story-telling where values and morals were imparted. Then we also learned that the smooth flow of a girl's whole life depended entirely upon her undergoing FGM so that refusing became as unthinkable as the dire future predicted for the child left unshorn. Indeed, no one ever talked about what could go wrong – and certainly not the extreme pain that segues into torture. Instead everything was meant to encourage us to accept the knife, abandoning resistance or fear. And so we, too, celebrated these amputations, viewing them as bestowing on initiates increased respect and enhanced status. Showered with numerous gifts, the graduate, no longer a child, would have become a woman and an asset to the group.

Festivities for kids

During the ceremonies, we young children would be allowed to eat, feast and dance to the traditional jig whose text lauded and praised the courageous who have just been cut. Ironically, beforehand, we were never permitted anywhere near the 'circumcision' rooms where screams would surely have frightened us away. Nor were we allowed to visit the victims. Only after they had healed would we see them again. Otherwise, we would have known how inhumanely they had been treated. In fact, the older girls would be isolated on a different homestead far from uncircumcised children, to remain there until their bodies had mended and resumed normal function. To limit our interactions, the elders warned us that because these girls had now been turned into 'adults', they had become off limits to us kids. We were forbidden to mingle or play with them.

For you see, the 'circumcised' now belonged to a different, advanced 'age set'. Only after we too had confronted the razor would we be permitted to fool around, hang out, or take care of chores together. Our elders told us that girls who have been 'circumcised' now had a special 'status' and deserved to be treated differently -- better than the way we were treated. During recovery, they were prepared special meals, treats also promised to us once we had become candidates ourselves. Of course, this made us jealous. The favor showered on that season's 'chosen' made every child long for the blade.

All these efforts that shielded us from the harsh realities of the procedure pushed us to admire and even desire it. After all, who wouldn't want to enjoy the elevated social status that came with it?

To understand the psychology here, you must be aware that, as kids, we were systematically humiliated in ways I now know to have gone against children's rights. We were deceived by all means possible, tricked into loving a so-called 'good practice' because of its artificial 'positive' change. No one ever mentioned long-term negative effects. Only afterward did reality dawn on me, and I realized that, for the girl child, adverse consequences far outweigh anything good.

Whilst an adult is free to submit herself to the ritual, a child without formed judgment never 'consents'. She simply undergoes the mutilation (which in this case is irrevocable) while she is totally vulnerable. The child's rights are violated since children are not consulted nor given a choice about facing the knife. Instead, for years, their minds have been manipulated by the old women who want girls to think 'circumcision' is what they need most in their lives.

The custom banned, and yet ...

Despite Kenya's passage of The Children's Act of 2001 to protect the young from harmful cultural practices and the nation's president having condemned FGM in 1983, the practice goes on. Similarly, numerous NGOs and human rights activists excoriate FGM internationally and within Kenya as a violation of human rights, yet little progress has been made. FGM remains prevalent and requires a more integrated approach.

For in fact, the Children's Act of 2001, now in place for over a decade, has not prevented it. Its tenacious hold on tradition remains, especially among pastoral groups. And even worse, the elders of my community, in obvious defiance on hearing the edict, issued a statement to the authorities. Protesting that female 'circumcision' is a cultural right reserved exclusively by the tribe, they warned the central government that it had no business telling them to stop.

As a Maasai who knows all too well the effects of FGM, I feel obliged to tell not only the Maasai elders but the world about the harm girl children suffer, including me. When addressing Maasai in Kenya about my personal experience, I acknowledge that efforts to condemn the practice haven't worked. Quite the contrary. It appears to be spreading and the health risks as well. The rite had always been damaging, but now previously unknown diseases accompany it, such as sexually transmitted infections (STI's), HIV/AIDS and hepatitis, among others.

From my experience as a ten-year-old, I bear witness to the fact that FGM is not only traumatic but also perilous; it can bring life-long pain, suffering, and even death to girls. I would like to see the Maasai community conserve our rich culture. Let's keep rituals, feasting and blessings on initiates but stop – full stop! – cutting genitalia.

The significance of FGM to the Maasai community

As a Maasai, I have been raised to feel great respect for our culture, and although female 'circumcision' is claimed by some, even among us, to be an outdated practice, it remains difficult for many to leave a way of life and adopt a new one, especially since, thus far, Maasai customs as a whole have survived largely intact. If FGM were not so tightly woven into the traditional fabric, convincing us to stop might be easier. But this magnitude of change would seem possible only with patience over the long run. ...

I paused at this point in my writing, overcome by a sense of malaise, wondering how to address a tricky issue of pride. You'll agree, of course, that the Maasai regard female 'circumcision' differently from the rest of the world, but the fact that we practice it, I must insist, does not make us lesser people. Our traditional ways of thinking have taught us that FGM is positive; that it improves a child's life. From the Maasai perspective, then, the time-honored practice has the following aims.

A wrong rite of passage

The primary reason the Maasai give for FGM is its use as a rite of passage from immaturity to womanhood, making a girl ready for marriage. As you have already read, we young children were made to believe a 'circumcised' girl ripens, gains in obedience, and becomes aware of her role in the family and society as a whole. We also learn that once 'circumcised' we would enjoy the respect of our elders and peers since despite our tender years, we would no longer count as kids.

How, exactly, are these rewards presented?

Before the procedure, girls are brought together daily, inspired not to fear, and assured that the most heroic will reap the best gifts. Initiates are also told that young men and their families will be watching and select wives only from among the most courageous. Thus, aspiration to be chosen by influence and wealth creates devotees of the ordeal. My feeling was that stakes like these propelled FGM beyond the status of a mere tradition; instead, as a lifestyle, its culmination in a show of heroism would also make me a hero for life. After all, the cutting isn't even the most spectacular of the day's events. Rather, festivities are boundless, and the whole village celebrates a girl's passage to maturity, her accession to another level of existence.

Now, parents make most decisions, but in some cases girls beg to be 'done' earlier, giving in to peer pressure, ridicule and insults. Elders would warn those just circumcised to remain steadfast. "Don't ever reveal your ordeal," they were told. Instead, they were exhorted to motivate us to face the knife in silence, as they, ideally, had done. So whenever we asked them, "What was it like?" they would lie. "It was fine," they'd say. "Everything's ok," and push us away. They would show us the gifts they had received and describe how everyone was ululating, dancing and praising them for their great achievement. They would also mock us and call us 'babies' because we had not yet confronted what they had. It was even more hurtful because girls we used to play with were now telling us to get lost. "Babies like you are beneath us," they scoffed.

Sadly, their strategy worked. Most of us felt irritated enough to swear to join in the following season, but really, all we wanted was to escape the taunting and humiliation.

In the past, Maasai girls had been 'circumcised' at 17 or 18 years old, the age when a girl was considered ready for marriage. But now, victims are between 8 and 15. Why? The trend can be attributed to parental worry about girls becoming sexually active, sometimes as young as ten, thus increasing the risk of pregnancy before being cut – a community taboo.

Furthermore, the clitoris itself is blamed. Considered an aggressive appendage, local belief holds that it threatens the male organ and even endangers babies during delivery. How are neonates imperiled? The baby's head touching the mother's clitoris will, it is thought, lower the child's IQ. Consequently, villagers consider the girl with a clitoris 'unclean' and unmarriageable. Anyone keeping her genital intact poses a threat, ultimately fatal to a man whose manhood might brush against her clit. In fact, so dangerous does she appear that the Council of Elders has passed a ruling: pregnancy before 'circumcision' makes the girl an outcast ineligible ever to marry in the tribe. Her choices are restricted to men from other groups. So, partly to prevent such tragic consequences of promiscuity, candidates for cutting are less often teens and more likely to be increasingly younger girls.

Another reason, however, for the cut is poverty. Because dowry can change hands only after 'circumcision', no matter the age of the betrothed, parents book their girls off for marriage to start receiving the bride price. The amputation tells suitors when to start instalments which, once paid up, entitle them to come and get their spouse. This is done in an orderly manner giving the mother time to teach the (too) young intended how to treat a man. And even if already wedded, the teen can remain in her parents' home for as long as five more years.

Still another motive behind the downward trend in age is that children under ten are hardly old enough to refuse nor strong enough to resist. At the same time, they are coming increasingly to know their rights, and maybe a hint of insipient rebellion is also making initiates younger.

For parents have begun to apply an ironic and misguided viewpoint; they contend that smaller kids suffer fewer traumas. Whether true or not, escaping notice is important as well, for, as we have seen, the government made FGM illegal under the Children's Act of 2001.

What really baffles me is how aware I am of just such motives, older people seducing children into undergoing rites of passage whose actual benefit accrues to the grown-ups in the form of wealth. Offspring bear the consequences since whatever they go through violates children's rights including their right to health, freedom, security and protection.

Psychological damage and lost childhoods

Prematurely declaring a child's entrance into womanhood has several negative results. A form of sexual abuse, it exposes the girl to knowledge beyond what is age-appropriate. Too young to understand the essence of what she is being pushed into, she cannot give true consent. With her brain still young, she should be educated, not cut. When hindered from growing into adulthood both mentally and physically, she ends up missing out on vital stages of development including formal education in schools.

Once 'circumcised', initiates are no longer viewed as little kids. Despite continuing to behave like youngsters, they are forced to adopt an adult mien. This makes FGM an ineffective rite of passage that merely 'marks' the child's body as grown-up while she remains physically and mentally a minor. In fact, because most cut girls still want to play, mingle with and dress like their age-mates, and conduct themselves like intact children, they can end up isolated and depressed. They may also feel resentful of a society that, to fulfill its own purpose, has neglected and used them.

Let's be frank about this. Once married, they experience unwanted sexual contact and this in turn can seem like torture because it so far exceeds what their childhood can bear. Just consider how many girls below 15, too young to face the responsibilities of wives, run away from husbands. At this age they should be playing, schooling and engaging in age-appropriate social duties.

All this may seem obvious to you and, indeed, to most readers, but a true hindrance to abolition is the practical collusion of the girls. The importance and seriousness accorded to the ceremony have always had an impact on children's thinking. While still small, you understand that 'circumcision' is a major event that everyone respects. As already mentioned, my friends and I believed that FGM was essential to our lives – and that no one could ever be successful without it. They preach that only a cut girl will receive gifts, marry well and have wealth brought to her parents to enable family stability. In other words, girls are taught to value FGM more than education. Thus, thinking that marriage, not schooling, will bring fortune, many pupils drop out for 'circumcision'.

To preserve sexual morality in girls

If you ask them, the Maasai will assure you that the rite reduces a girl's desire for sex, making her less avid for pre-marital intercourse. Dispensing with the clitoris is thought to curb sexual activity before, and ensure fidelity within, the conjugal relationship. And elders are quick to point to neighboring communities whose uncut girls, freer with their bodies, reap their just rewards for promiscuity in elevated cases of HIV and AIDS.

But really! Does a ten-year-old experience sexual desire for a penis? Does she want, frankly, penetration? Is she the one initiating sex? Not according to my point of view. Sex happens when an older male lures or forces her into cooperating for HIS pleasure, not hers, and she should therefore not be blamed. The guilt is his. More attention should be shifted to major causes of early sexuality other than bodily desires of girls. Blaming girls for men's selfish lust is male chauvinism 101.

This is true whether the male partner is old or young. Teen boys, too, seduce or coerce adolescent girls. Excising a child's genitals to prevent the consequences is discrimination pure and simple. Sex education for both girls and boys promises a far better solution to the problem of early sexuality.

Society focuses too much on the sexuality of teenage females anyway. Parents have always concentrated on the sexual life of the girl, including her marriage, and turn a blind eye to other important aspects of her life such as personal interests and education. Considering the cut more important than learning, guardians withdraw their daughter from school, thereby denying the child her right to education. How does this necessarily follow? Losing the clitoris changes her entire life. Sadly, in many cases, she, too, no longer finds scholarship important, having been taught to behave like a wife – even though she is far too young!

Considering FGM as a means to preserve girls' sexual morality is truly short-sighted, not to mention illogical. OK. Let's grant that trauma in the most sensitive part of the vulva can be expected to temper the urge to have sex. But what happens later, when she is married? No one says they intend to make sexual experience within marriage miserable, but that's the result. In practical terms, then, add to denial of the right to education denial of the right to enjoy sex when the child grows up.

Upholding our cultural tradition

As I have said, the Maasai community regards 'circumcision' not as a religious but as a cultural practice that elevates a person from childhood to adulthood and must be performed if a girl is to become an adult. In this sense, the rite serves as an integral part of the Maasai peoples' way of life.

For many Maasai, therefore, no reason is needed beyond the fact that it has always been done. In the words of some elders: "We were born and found our people practicing it, so we just follow the culture in place. No one asks whether or not the girl should be cut – this is like the law of the land, almost impossible to avoid." As a child, I was told by my mother, "Female 'circumcision' is our culture.

Because we were born into it, we shouldn't be forced to abandon it, an act that would annoy our ancestors and curse the whole community. Those who dislike it would do better to tell us how to improve the procedure rather than stop it. Why should we be forced to adopt a culture not our own?"

Thus, Maasai attachment to tradition – and convinced that 'circumcision' belongs to this inheritance – weakens efforts to discourage the practice. Opposition is perceived as diluting or "kill-ing" the culture. This concern was raised by the Council of Elders as they wondered why the government and other players were attempting to eradicate FGM. And the atti-tude is not that of seniors alone. Even younger Maasai think FGM is a significant aspect of their culture making its assaults on health irrelevant.

So what do I say to all this? I find it disturbing that society should concentrate on culture while ignoring deleterious effects on those it harms. The focus on pleasing ancestors ignores the welfare of children. Education is needed: those who favor FGM should be made to understand that what counts as culture should not oppress and torture girls, robbing them of childhoods. If only the attention brought to 'culture' were di-verted to education, we'd have already made FGM history.

Why has this *not* been done? If life is dynamic and so is culture, you would expect to find some waning of tradition. This is in fact the case, for unlike today, the past witnessed even higher percentages of cut female members of the tribe. Perhaps acceptance then and lower tolerance now are related to rising awareness of complications linked to the procedure that had been entirely missing. Then as well, supposing that complex diseases transmitted by shared knives existed, – like AIDS –, they weren't recognized as such. Today, at last, knowledge of health risks is growing coupled with a shrinking number of excisers whose age, weakness, and inability to train successors augurs well for an end to the rite.

Economic motives

Underestimated in abolition efforts is, in my opinion, the economic motive. Quite simply, an uncircumcised girl fetches a lower bride price.

While for some Maasai FGM is as integral to our culture as naming children after relatives, others use it to increase their wealth. The latter self-interest reigns among pastoral communities where the number of animals a man has determines his wealth and wins him respect. No wonder he books his girls early to be married off in exchange for more cattle and goats. Among the Maasai, only a 'circumcised' girl is worth booking for marriage so the parents can, as already mentioned, start receiving dowry.

Understanding the dynamic here depends on recognizing the importance of bride price where FGM persists. A deeply entrenched custom, bride-price means that any girl who refuses 'circumcision' undermines the would-be wealth her father expects on her betrothal.

Before judging, however, and to be fair, you must take poverty into account. The stakes can be truly dire. Many Maasai families cannot afford to give their children formal schooling, so, to spare them hunger, they want them wed young. Because Maasai girls are traditionally considered children until cut, and therefore unsuitable brides, FGM remains a prerequisite to marriage. Due to such deeply intertwined cultural beliefs, families go to great lengths to 'circumcise'.

But by definition, aren't a child's rights abused when society places a material value – an explicit, if negotiable price tag – on a girl? When they say that a cut girl will fetch more bride price than an uncut one, they imply that the scar on the girl's body increases her material worth in her suitor's family's eyes. Based on the ancestral background of the girl's larger extended kin, several suitors' families approach the parents of the mutilated girl to express their interest in the daughter on behalf of their scion. Only then are they allowed to bid the amount of dowry they are willing to pay. The highest bidder is given the chance so that, in most cases, the wealthiest wins. The girl's folks also receive a guarantee, that their daughter shall be well fed (at least) and not starve.

In other cases, when her family has a sterling reputation, the daughter is booked even before she suffers FGM, and the groom pays to have her mutilated. In such cases the dowry can be much high-er than for later booking because other families have been denied the opportunity to express interest and make their bid. Here, since the family has already committed the child, ensuring her acceptability via 'circumcision' becomes even more pressing so that dowry payments can begin. You see how commercialized the practice has become, increasing young girls' vulnerability to FGM and compounding resistance to ending it.

Consequences for the child are, as I've already hinted, horrendous. Neither the young person's age nor her understanding count as a measure of maturity; adulthood is marked by the amputation of a body part. All this feeds into girls' low self-esteem, as they are denied experience and time to mature. And schooling falls by the wayside. As I've said before, the community would do better to focus on education, for learning promotes mental growth, creativity, and knowledge, enabling girls, like boys, to gain financial independence and thereby help alleviate their parents' suffering and poverty.

It further grieves me to know that this system opens my people to a specific form of censure: not only outsiders, but I, too, believe that valuing children in terms of wealth is inhumane. Circumstance, necessity and despair may play a role here, but using a child as a tool to fight poverty violates that child's right to freedom, to make choices, to get married, to determine when to marry, whom to marry or even not to marry at all. Presently, custom co-opts these real markers of maturity, especially when parents impose a husband on a girl without consideration for her feelings.

The Maasai defend FGM for other reasons as well, among them the conviction that no sensible wife could possibly possess a clitoris. The 'uncircumcised', it is argued, are immoral; they make rude

spouses and disrespectful daughters-in-law. Men, who firmly believe this is so, refuse to offer themselves as husbands to the uncut
– and the girls know it. I grew up under threat of being left out of
marriage altogether. Though I've said it in these pages many times
before, from a tender age it is drummed into us that no man will
propose if we remain intact.

I sometimes suspect that male tastes are behind hygienic and
aesthetic arguments for FGM, the belief that female genitalia are
ugly, malodorous and in need of enhancement by blade. If I were
to take the podium, I imagine myself telling the tribe: "It's unethical
to think that a girl is born 'ugly' and that beauty emerges only when
you cut her up. Every body part plays a role, and removing one means
certain malfunction. Please understand that we can clean ourselves
down there without your resorting to torture. After all, the scalpel
doesn't work as well as sex education would."

Of course, I've already spoken to peers and elders and noted with
dismay their inability to explain how FGM truly qualifies a child to become some older man's wife. What about maturity, responsibility
and love? Shouldn't wives exhibit these? Do these qualities count
for nothing? They certainly fade to the point of disappearing behind the one criterion that trumps all else: that the new bride must
be scarred.

If it were up to me, I'd teach my people about qualities to consider when choosing marriage partners – and the cut would not be
one of them! If I were a man, I would want an educated wife, not
a subordinate I had bought for dowry. Any man's refusal to marry
an intact girl reflects poorly on him for disrespecting children and
their rights. And if he really wants her brutal mutilation, what kind
of husband will he be? Will he continue his ruthless demands? Insist she obey? Make her suffer for his ego and his pleasure?

FGM is diabolical in that it causes a child to think like a man – to convince her he's right, and that the best she can imagine is serving him in marriage. Make her think that, when at seven, or ten, or even thirteen, a body part comes off, she's ready for wifehood. What about making her wholesome instead? Encouraging talents, nurturing skills, cultivating her mind – all that is left out.

How the Maasai perform FGM

Parents are the key decision-makers; whether a girl undergoes FGM or not is up to them. As we've seen, the older generation lures kids into wanting the cut by making them believe in the necessity and importance of the process, not only in the child's life but also in the community's. Let me tell such parents here, "You're most to blame." Efforts to end FGM shatter on the rock of parental resistance so the need for direct talk to parents is great.

Naturally, in some cases girls decide for themselves, but they are most often motivated from the outside by peer pressure or classmates' mockery. Their guardians, mainly mothers, who could influence them otherwise, merely confirm the daughter's choice and manage the affair. In our particular clan, more women than men, and especially elderly women, are involved, truly ironic and unfair to the child who expects protection from caregivers, not torture and humiliation. Yet too often you will find them witnessing their daughter's mutilation, a perceived betrayal that leads many girls to feel insecure even in their own homes. Parents thus deny their children the right to protection, health, and freedom.

As for the men who, as we have seen, demand shorn brides, often they can't even tell whether their betrothed is 'circumcised' or not but depend on the assurance of female witnesses. The child's mother is usually on hand to certify that the cut is as it should be, another indication of parental ignorance and selfishness, because the main concern is not the daughter's well-being but satisfaction for the suitor in anticipation of dowry installments. Once again we see child abuse condoned by conventions that hold wealth and family above the safety of the child.

Among the Maasai, FGM is generally carried out by the elderly (most often but not exclusively women) assigned to this task or by traditional birth attendants paid by the girls' suitors or her family, in money or in kind. What exactly qualifies these excisers cannot be explained. People trust them, however, with their children's health, their respect based on the practitioner's wisdom and seniority but certainly not on formal medical training since, generally, there is none. These lay medics carry out a complex procedure on a delicate organ yet have no clinical background since they never attended medical school. No wonder that girls' lives are at risk and are even sometimes lost.

Instruments include special knives, broken glass, or razorblades, depending on the 'circumciser', although a scalpel or scissors may have been obtained. Sometimes the tools are new but more often are not; they may have served other purposes or pierced the skin of other 'patients'. Seldom sterilized by traditional operators, the inventory also comprises suturing items like sewing needles, domestic thread or pre-selected nylon fiber. These items' nature and quality reinforce the image of deficient medical knowledge on the part of the cutter and pose a clear threat to victims' lives.

The lack of hygiene is compounded by the absence of surgical gloves or sanitary hands. And even when soap is used, moisture can make trouble, too. After all, wet fingers are slippery and, should the operator have difficulty pinching the clitoris or the skin being removed, she may well dry herself on the girl's thighs or even in the sand, thus improving dexterity in grabbing the clitoris but increasing the risk of infection. Also amplifying danger is the custom among some circumcisers who use their long nails as pincers. Nor are rings, amulets and other ornaments generally removed, as these items are not viewed by the traditional health worker as likely sources of contamination. Again, all this imperils the child.

Since bleeding will occur and secretions follow for some days, the family usually finds an old mat or floor covering that can later be discarded. Sometimes sand is placed on the mat under the victim's buttocks to absorb blood and other fluids. It is not unheard of among more affluent or educated families, aware of the risks of infection, to provide clean sheets and cotton wool, but this is a rare scenario among the Maasai. Consider, too, the risk inherent in ill-constructed Maasai houses, called *manyattas*, which are poorly ventilated with inadequate lighting since they have no windows or louvers and only a single door. A faulty 'operating theatre' can, in turn, compound the likelihood of injury and infection.

Furthermore, the Maasai celebrate female 'circumcision' as a communal and public occasion, held during a specified period determined by community elders. The cutting ceremonies are colorful events, marked by public dancing, drinking and feasting. Although a girl is excised inside the *manyatta*, an audience gathers outside in an open field with the elders present. Traditional songs contain messages urging courage and exhorting those who have not yet faced the knife to be ready for the next cutting season. Individual families organize coaching sessions on married life, usually by relatives, for their own initiates immediately after the procedure.

The power of community leaders in upholding traditions in all clans in Maasai land should not be underestimated. FGM, for instance, takes place when the Council of Elders says it does. Traditionally, though, it has been scheduled towards the end of each year's rainy season when the land provides plenty of pasture and water for the animals so even the herders may be present. The herds, too, healthy and fat, have enjoyed ample pasture and provide in turn the high quantities and quality of meat, milk and blood needed for the public festival.

This particular schedule also reveals a humane belief: that the dry season following the rainy one allows injuries to heal faster with less pain. The rainy season, it is thought, increases the wounds' torment, slows recovery, and increases the risk of infection as a result of the cold. Moreover, herbs to aid recovery that need moisture to sprout mature in time to medicate the cuts.

Another option is December when the holiday is long, the girls are home, and they have weeks to heal.

Nonetheless, 'circumcision' can take place at any time throughout the year, and some parents have been known to remove pupils from class, evidence that the procedure trumps education, present and future. Some of the freshly wounded, too distracted to concentrate on homework, take long before they return to school, while others withdraw completely, their formal learning now effectively over. In contrast, girls fortunate to have their school curriculum teach about FGM know what to expect. Should they wish to resist, however, there's only one choice -- to flee.

Surprisingly, despite a high rate of illiteracy, most community members know about the Act outlawing FGM but continue the practice in secret to escape prosecution. Considering FGM to be a family affair, they feel that issues and matters relating to it fall not to the government but to the tribe. Now, as we have seen, this had not been traditionally so. Festivities had been extravagantly public. But this proprietary attitude accounts for a significant change in the way things are run now and for the challenges in implementing the 2001 Children's Act, for no matter what the dispute, police and the courts are avoided.

Privatization of FGM among the Maasai is therefore becoming the norm. As schools and other public fora raise awareness, -- religious organizations, for instance, integrate children's rights into sermons and pastoral lessons--, and local administration reluctantly implements the 2001 Children's Act, FGM is transformed from an outdoor to an indoor event. To escape activists' eyes, public cutting ceremonies and festivities are fading. The practice has become increasingly secretive, although sometimes, a tightknit group of families may have their daughters 'circumcised' together. The cover-ups, however, are not yet water-tight. Suspicion may be aroused, for example, when initiates show off their new-bought clothes and shoes, or when, if well-off, they mention special treatment and better food.

If traditional birth attendants or, at times, nurses remain, as before, the practitioners of choice, the venue has changed. Increasing numbers operate in the girls' own homes while wealthier youth find themselves in clinical surroundings, in the hospital or health center where qualified medical practitioners earn extra cash. Arrangements are made discreetly, and hospitals charge between 500-2000 Kenyan shillings, depending on "market rates." For the traditional birth attendant, payment is made in goats or cows, and the cut girls' families pay.

All this is very sad, because children go on suffering the outrage of amputation despite efforts by government, civil society organizations and angry individuals like me to spare them – as I, an injured girl, would love to have been spared. As much as I resist concluding that our efforts have been fruitless, Maasai who defy the law, continue mutilating in their homes or clinics, and simply refuse to stop throw us an immense challenge. No obstacles, nothing meant to discourage them, seems to have worked.

Let's just say that I'm as stubborn as they are, with determination and a fighting spirit. I want FGM to end, and I'll do all I can to see that Maasai girls, like the child I was, are kept from such unspeakable, degrading pain. The new face of Maasai youth is mine – an inspiration and a source of hope for healthy and whole generations to come. We *will* eliminate this harmful traditional practice.

The cut itself – what happens ...

The Maasai practice clitoridectomy, excising the visible part of the clitoris and at times the adjacent labia followed at times by stitching – my case.

Very early morning provides the most auspicious hour because, it is believed, the dawn's coolness minimizes bleeding and pain. Despite being awakened unusually early, however, girls generally don't suspect what awaits them. Preparations are kept secret until everything is in place. Why? People will answer with surprising frankness: to obviate hiding or running away.

On that morning when my turn came, without breakfast, we girls were made to remove our clothes and face the chill, the idea being that the cold would numb us. Then, after we were shaved clean and our bodies covered in red soil, we were given shoes made of cows' hide to wear. On the previous evening, someone had milked a cow, added water and left the liquid to stay overnight. The following day, to anesthetize us further, the mixture would be poured all over us.

And then, the moment came.

I was made to lie down at a slant; varied postures depend on the girl's age and strength to resist. They would have bigger girls squat on a stool or mat facing the circumciser at a convenient height offering a clear view of the incisive part. These accommodations benefit the excisers, usually the elderly whose sight may be impaired and who may find bending over difficult.

Following the command to strip, we were told to lie down. Hardly had I hit the ground than my thighs were seized by two adults who yanked them apart, crushing my hips. A third person's weight descended on my head and chest. To prevent kicks, they bent my legs at the knee, tied them at the ankles and extended the rope to my thighs. Two more women imprisoned my hands. Clearly, they presumed I'd fight.

Then, without missing a beat, the circumciser grabbed my clitoris, pinched it between her unclean nails and, – slash! – cut it off. She then presented the severed organ to senior female relatives for judgment: had sufficient flesh been removed? Was one knife thrust enough or were more required? In the makeshift clinic– a *man-yatta* like the others–, my ear-splitting shrieks and heavy bleeding seemed not to have moved the auditors at all. And yes, this time, one whack had done the trick. Others wouldn't be so 'lucky'.

Now, with the offending organ chopped, the jury ululated, and the 'circumciser' proceeded to slice off the labia minora. This had now become a messy business as by then I was blaring, writhing, and bleeding in torrents so that, armed with no more than fingers and nails, the torturer barely captured the elusive liquid skin.

But after an eternity, the wounding was complete. Sufficient flesh had been ablated to permit the desired fusion. Next of course, the injury required aftercare. It is strongly believed that the traumatized tissue should not be left to nature but helped along, not only to prevent more cutting but also to ensure the exciser's repute. Failed recuperation would damage her standing and discourage clients.

Thus to hasten healing, the operator readied the lesion for stitching by juxtaposing the raw edges of the labia majora where she had confiscated skin and, with needle and nylon, made a tight seam. (Lacking thread, thorns may be inserted instead and, like lacing a shoe, a string wound around the hooks.)

Next, the exciser broke a raw egg on the wound and sprinkled it with herbs so that the brew, augmented by my blood, could crust ...

Though certainly not universally effective, the concoction was supposed to prevent bacterial infection and, in any case, it was the only prophylactic.

To ascertain that the urethra has not been accidentally closed, either by blood clot or suture, I was encouraged to urinate a few hours later which luckily I did successfully but under a lot of pain.

Then the circumciser, in symbolic ritual, blessed me. "...You are now grown up," she said. "You should not die married to one man, but marry many men in future..." Outside the ritual house, men were singing and dancing in agreement and they, too, acknowledged my achievement, encouraging me never to die with one man.

Frankly, I was unimpressed, in too much pain to care. I was glad that it was over, but it really wasn't; the aftermath is nearly as excruciating as the prelude. Healing requires immobility.

To prevent movement my legs were bound together from hip to toe and I was ordered to lie on my side. Despite lack of antiseptic for the wound, I was tied up for a week. Only then were the bindings slightly loosened and I was allowed to take small steps. On the seventh day, the sutures were removed and the thorns, too, provided that the circumciser finds the labial fusion satisfactory. The leg straps then disappear after another week.

As for the instruments of torture, the exciser washed the knife with cold water to prevent rust on the blade, applied skimmed fat from cow's milk, tied it with a piece of cloth and stored it in unsanitary conditions to wait for the next season. The tool would emerge for use on other young girls, without being sterilized in the meantime, thus increasing the risk of infection, lockjaw from rust, or transmission of contagious diseases.

So how did I *feel* during all this? My tone in the telling has been calm, but I wasn't tranquil at all. The so-called anesthetic herbs didn't work. In fact the whole healing process was torture in itself. Just imagine having your legs bound, confined to a single position unable to budge. I found it really hard. Moreover, since we were isolated so the younger girls wouldn't see us and run off when their turn came, we suffered severe loneliness. I felt abandoned and longed to be cared for. And there were no distractions. Yesterday's playmates were now lost to us.

Among the many regrettable aspects of our treatment, I find the trickery hardest to swallow. In so many ways we were deceived! Why had the elders hidden everything from us? Yes, I know, to prevent our objections. But if they feared we would bolt, then something wasn't right, was it? They, too, sensed it. And once we girls realized what catastrophe was about to ensue, when the news broke only on the morning of the trauma, we were truly shocked, fearful, abject and hopeless. The experience was horrible but no one seemed to care about our feelings. No one cared how I felt at home beforehand, exposed to cruel treatment with no relative to rescue me. No one cared how I felt naked in the morning chill, my body trembling from cold. Expected to conduct ourselves with courage and maturity, maybe we could have done so if only we'd understood why! Why were we being shaved? Why covered in red soil? Why were our bodies in such great pain while songs and dances filled the air, and above all, why were we being praised? It made no sense.

Of course, growing up in a cutting culture you have an inkling of what lies ahead. But you've been convinced it's good.

It's not. It's a scam. Never had anyone mentioned how brutal it is.

So I sobbed and wept and bawled ... If the whole world was against me, why not rage and curse the ones who had held me down?

They had caused this agony in urination, acid in contact with an open wound. But you had to pee to prevent much worse. What if the urethra closed? You'd go under the blade again. So you bit your lip as the liquid dripped.

Seventeen years have passed but not a single second of emotional time. All that I have just described is indelible in my mind. They wanted to humiliate me, but I've defied them in the aftermath, or at least tried to shed the worst effects of the inhumane abuse of FGM. They 'blessed' me by wishing me a life with many men? Well, what about HIV and AIDS? They considered me at ten years old mature and ready to be booked for marriage so my parents could receive the payments?

I have escaped to Germany, but knowing how many other girls have not breaks my heart.

Risk and trauma: Physical

Although from one instance to the next, cutting among the Maasai can diverge slightly from what I have just described, all forms produce deleterious effects on physical health. Consequences that begin immediately can be grouped into both long- and short-term which manifest within a period extending from a few hours after ablation to ten days later. Long-term complications are life-long, can be irreversible and require medical attention. Sadly, however, lack of access to health facilities, stigma and ignorance of the cause of their distress prevent most girls from consulting a clinician.

To begin with immediate complications, the event itself is highly traumatic for a child. Naked force is used: the women who restrained me and my legs exerted considerable pressure and I was fearful to the point of panic. Cutting the clitoral root made me instantly weak and powerless, leaving a certain residue of impotence that has haunted me for the rest of my life. The pain, too, was extreme, in the total absence of anesthetics and antiseptics, and I bled profusely because, as I found out later, the clitoral artery had been hit. The bleeding which led at first to shock then turned into anemia. But at least in one respect, I was lucky. Though my bleeding was heavy, I didn't hemorrhage and die from loss of blood.

An infection got me, though, likely caused by septic instruments in an unhygienic space. Fortunate to be alive, I nonetheless suffered from pelvic inflammation and might have contracted blood poisoning or tetanus which, had these conditions remained untreated, could have sealed my fate like that of too many others. I risked HIV and hepatitis as well, because a single tool maimed many. Despite knowledge that one blade for a troop of children brings these risks, conditions that prevail in hiding increase the likelihood of a minimum number of blades.

So you see, if fortune kept me free of AIDS, it didn't prevent infection. And although, unlike girls wounded by inept practitioners, my bladder and urethra were untouched, I suffered urinary retention from fear of excruciating pain while voiding. Not only when urine comes in contact with the wound does the torture ensue, but intense discomfort can also result from tissue swelling and urethral injury. And I've lost track of the number of urinary tract infections. It seems as though the affliction visited us all.

Well, you're probably thinking you've heard enough by this time.

Not yet, I'm afraid. Even more troublesome customs follow.

Once the aforementioned herbal concoction was applied to the wound, we were forbidden to bathe before it had healed completely. Why? We were told that liquid might promote infection so that, kept dry, the excision would mend faster. So for two *l o n g* weeks washing was out, despite the red soil and blood stains on our bodies, and they became messier and smellier day by day. In great discomfort, I got itchy rashes around the vagina and skin infections due to the dirt and sweat.

Regarding the nearly ubiquitous urinary tract infections, FGM victims remain prone to them long after the actual excision, and these inflammations are not innocent. They have been known to lead to kidney failure.

In 2007 in my community, Narok, Kenya, a mother organized 'circumcision' for her six-year-old against the husband's wish. The angered father, too late to rescue the child, took her away afterward and had her stay with an aunt in Nairobi. Four years later, when the girl returned to Narok, her grandmother, convinced the initial cutting had been insufficient, had her done a second time. The girl, who has since developed kidney problems because she can never pass urine properly, visits the dialysis clinic every three weeks. The parents have apologized to her and have never cut her sisters – but that hardly makes for a truly happy ending. ...

Risk and trauma: emotional and psychological

FGM can leave a lasting mark on the life and mind of those who endure it. In fact, of all side-effects of FGM, the mental and emotional residues last longest. My own childhood experience has left me with two psychological conditions from which I suffer.

The first is an "anxiety state" originating from lack of sleep and hallucinations, and these in turn correlate with PTSD, since the trauma imposed by such a practice easily compares to torture. When five adults overpower a slim ten-year-old, she reacts with panic and then, from unspeakable pain, with shock. The practice produces horror, and re-running the indelible script has led to white nights the moment the scenario flashes through my mind. Oh, how I wish I could forget that old woman lowering her knife on me, chopping something off, and provoking a torrent of blood. How I'd love to disremember!

But since I was ten, when it happened, it hasn't left me. Sleep leads to nightmares that wake me up to weep.

Remembering the "good stories" we always heard about FGM does not comfort me. It reinforces the deceit.

The second psychological condition is "reaction depression," a result of delayed healing which in my case was a complicated matter. To start, the stress triggered behavioural disturbances in me closely linked to loss of confidence in care givers – including my own mother. When she entered the room to confirm her satisfaction, I felt helpless and betrayed. Aware that she had simply stood by and watched me writhe in agony, I not only lost trust in her but also, worse, I felt hatred. My mother, someone who should have protected me from such brutality, had done nothing. Yes, I blamed her, and kept on blaming her for failure to intervene, and I remained acutely conscious that she had instigated it; she had arranged for this mind-breaking event. And she did it, as most do, for her own material interest without caring about my well-being. This, at least, is what I knew as a child, and the judgment has stayed with me until now.

Initiates' isolation on a different homestead was also mentally disturbing. While nursing painful wounds, we were kept away from family.

I remember a cosmic solitude. With bound legs and no friends to interact and play with, my stress and agitation grew. How did this differ from abduction? And what about my rights, I think now at a distance of some years, to liberty and freedom from torture?

Yes, the so-called 'healing' proceeded apace, but stress remained in strained family relations. Those I loved most in my life, I now 'knew', were against me. Had they not allowed, even approved, what had happened to me? Then clearly they no longer loved me, and so from then on, having lost all trust in them, I kept my problems locked inside. But no one could ever take their place and I have lived till now without a confidante, someone with whom to share the excruciating experience I had had.

FGM violates human rights

I wonder whether we don't have an instinct for human rights, since I never needed the UN to tell me that what had happened to me violated them.

But perpetrators clearly need reminding, so the UN has declared FGM in violation of the girl child's human rights. In that international body's official formulation, FGM contravenes the child's entitlement to the highest attainable standards of health; to be free of violence; and her right to life when stalked by death. It also infringes on the child's mental and physical integrity, in part by discriminating against her on the basis of sex; and it clearly flouts the child's right to be free from "cruel, inhuman, and degrading treatment."[2] The force and fury I went through identify FGM as torture.

Female Genital Mutilation violates human rights

I welcome provisions in several international instruments, even if they failed to rescue me.

The Universal Declaration of Human Rights (UDHR), an international convention that obligates Kenya, a signing state party, to follow its mandate includes children. Implicitly, they, too, benefit from concepts of dignity and the equal and inalienable rights of all members of the human family, in turn the cornerstone of freedom, justice and peace in the world. Yes, I am saying that, in the broadest sense, world peace is at stake in our fight to end FGM, and if Kenya is to promote full implementation of the pledge, it must support these rights and freedoms.

As a violation of children's rights, FGM breaches the following articles as laid down in the convention:

Article 3 states that we all have a right to life, freedom of choice and security. Now, even when FGM is carried out 'properly' by an experienced practitioner, – that is, it hasn't been a truly botched job –, it can still kill. Doing it always entails risk and is therefore always in violation of the Declaration of Human Rights.

Moreover, the child's decision is never truly her own, even if bullying makes her think so. As in my case, an assumption was made that I'd agreed implicitly based on the false information I'd been fed. When the moment came, however, I was impotent with no one to turn to for help. And let me assure you, I wanted OUT.

FGM also violates Article 5 of the Declaration: "No one shall be subjected to torture or to cruel, inhuman or degrading treatment or punishment."[3] Forcing someone to endure acute mental or physical pain, such as I suffered, is forbidden, and as you have seen, cutting is torture. The torment inflicted on me by both the clitoridectomy and the stitching – unbearable anguish – can hardly be expressed, and for days afterward, urinating only increased my wretchedness. Furthermore, removing a healthy clitoris also amounts to degrading treatment, for it only makes any kind of perverted sense at all if the organ in question, and hence its possessor, already lacks equality. Where female genitalia are demonized, so is the female, and slander of this type is degrading.

Article 16 (1 & 2) is also relevant. It states that all human beings despite their social background have the right to marry and found a family. And as for Maasai custom, paragraph 2 holds enhanced significance: "Marriage shall be entered into only with the free and full consent of the intending spouses." As we have seen, 'circumcising' a young girl means she is soon to be booked for marriage by parents more concerned with material gain than their daughter's happiness. This in turn denies the girl her right to enjoy marriage at the right time in the future, should she want to, and certainly infringes on her right never to marry at all. The imposition of marriage, which in the case of the under-aged is legalized rape, also indubitably damages physical and mental health.

The Declaration has anticipated this in Article 25 (1) concerning the human right to health and a certain minimum level of prosperity. "Everyone has the right to a standard of living adequate for … health and well-being … including food, clothing, housing, medical care and necessary social services…" FGM clearly denies victims their maxi-mum health and well-being by exposing them to the curses we have already seen: blockage of the urethra, recurrent urinary tract infections, tetanus, hepatitis, and other inflammations that easily lead to chronic suffering, disability and, possibly, sterility.

These cumulative handicaps, successfully resisted as they may be by many strong, self-confident 'circumcised' women, nonetheless contribute to a less than optimal school experience, but the right to learn has also been recognized and enshrined in the Declaration. Article 26 (1) states: "Everyone has the right to [free, compulsory, elementary] education…" And even more impressive is paragraph 2:

Education should be directed to the full development of the human personality and to the strengthening of respect for human rights and fundamental freedoms. It shall promote understanding, tolerance and friendship among all nations, racial or religious groups and shall further the activities of the United Nations for the maintenance of peace.[4]

The road to realizing these broad aims is strewn with landmines for the cut girl. Too often, once maimed, she drops out – of her own volition or parents' command as they have had her trimmed to accelerate the wedding and bring them wealth. Based on what I know, it appears that too many parents find FGM more valuable than education. And, sadly, the girls themselves follow their elders' lead. For initiates are told they have now become 'women' and if 'women', how can they possibly share a classroom with small kids? A false sense of pride thus keeps them home.

Children's rights

Because most FGM affects females younger than 18, – victims cluster between 5 and 15 years –, excision falls under the purview of children's rights. In addition to protections guaranteed, if not yet enforced, by signatories to the UN Declaration just discussed, additional international and local instruments apply.

The Convention on the Rights of the Child (CRC) (GA resolution 44/25 of 20 November 1989, entered into force 2 September 1990) and the African Charter on the Rights and Welfare of the Child (ACRWC) (ratified in November 2010 and signed by all but 8 member states of the African Union) set out the rights children should enjoy at every age, including especially what they need to thrive, – education, security and health –, and what they must be spared: violence, abuse and torture.

FGM violates a number of rights as laid down in these instruments. First, part 1, Article 2 of the CRC forbids discrimination based on the child's social, cultural or economic background. Now, discrimination is a broad concept and generally suggests exclusions, for instance with regard to housing (in the U.S. racially restrictive covenants used to prevent home purchase by black people, supported by banks' influence on 'redlining' districts to exclude them), professions (for instance, want ads by gender), or segregation and apartheid. But here I find evidence of bias experienced by a child within the context of FGM. For example, wasn't it discriminatory when, after my body was cut, I was forcibly cut off from my former friends? Remember that the blade that amputates a clitoris also separates the child from the adult. It throws away the clock, so to speak, since processes that should evolve – friendships, maturation – are violently displaced. A girl without her clitoris is defined as an adult subject to rules governing mature conduct. And adults in our culture do not play with children.

Discrimination also occurs if the girl has the courage and strength to resist. She will be socially excluded and her family as well. If she defies the razor and runs away, she forfeits all hope of local marriage. The consensus holds, no man will consider an outcast an adequate partner. Community respect with be withheld; the parents must bid good-bye to any dowry, and the dearth of suitors translates to bias against the uncut girl. FGM embeds itself in this web of cause and consequence.

Granted, this intolerance can generally be surmounted. It is not fatal. But many aspects of FGM can be deadly, so that whenever it's imposed, it violates Article 6 (1) of the CRC guaranteeing the right to life itself. Thus, in Article 6 (2), states are enjoined to restrict all activities or practices that may jeopardize a child's longevity. FGM is clearly implied, and as we have seen, health risks, even potentially mortal ones, abound. I won't catalogue here what's already been said, but add a few complicating factors: long-term danger may not be noticed in the early stages after mutilation; too many girls have little access to health facilities; and those that do are often young, embarrassed, frightened or too ill to make use of them. For innocent failure to take preventive steps, too many young women die.

Naturally, the right to life is more clearly violated when the link to cutting is direct. The girl's struggles, exciser's eyesight, inadequate lighting, and fragile immune systems – all these may occasion horrendous complications including excessive bleeding which can lead to anemia; blockage of the bladder which can lead to kidney failure; injury to the vulva that may prolong childbirth and lead not to one but two deaths, of the mother and her baby.

The African Charter on the Rights and Welfare of the Child (ACRWC) in Article 5 (1 & 2) reinforces the promise to defend the right to life. Kenya has signed, accepting the responsibility spelled out in Part 2, to ensure children maximum protection and opportunities to develop – a commitment clearly incompatible with government tolerance for FGM.

Equally indisputable is the violation by FGM of Article 19 (1) of the CRC which protects against mental and physical violence including maltreatment supposedly justified by traditional cultural practices. Signatory states have agreed to take all possible measures to ensure children's safety while in the care of their legal guardians. Because parents play such a key role in arranging for a daughter's 'ceremony', Article 19 provides for their censure.

Like the CRC, the ACRWC (African Charter), in Article 21 (1), reiterates commitment to oppose harmful social and cultural practices that may negatively affect a child throughout her life. Her welfare and dignity should not be jeopardized by FGM.

Excision is not, of course, the only hazard; the practice participates in a discriminatory pattern that includes child marriage. As mandated in Article 21 of the ACRWC, elevating the age of majority to 18 years is a step in the right direction for both of these human rights infringements. So is a mandatory registration of all new marriages by integrating respect for the law into customary life that in many respects disregards or defies it.

Even if the African Union were the only international unit with a special convention for child protection, this alone could answer African children's special need for consideration and defense. Child marriage, FGM, and a number of additional customs are dangerous – and this means treacherous vis-à-vis children's health. Article 24 (1, 2e, and 3) of the CRC guarantees the right to the highest attainable standard of health by placing healthcare under the purview of governments – a positive step not yet fully implemented even in wealthy Western nations (namely the USA). But the CRC enjoins African regimes to treat illness, facilitate rehabilitation, support basic health education, and teach nutrition – in sum, to provide both preventative and curative medical facilities and therapy. This commitment is obviously welcome because Article 3, on abolition of harmful traditional practices, makes combatting FGM of intrinsic value to the state. Eradicating FGM is in the state's self-interest, especially its economic interest. Mandated to spend money on health, regimes will want a rapid end to FGM.

Let's consider this in some detail. How much does it cost when young girls haemorrhage, as I nearly did, or grow anemic, become infected, run high fevers, need emergency care, or become chronic patients? Remember those unsterile instruments? And what about childbirth? How much extra will it cost to ensure the safety of neonates and mothers? And what about lost productivity? The loss to development as a whole? These sums are considerable, surely.

So let's review. The CRC is most concerned that everyone, in the public sector or a private home, behaves "in the best interests of the child." Is her best interest served by deceiving her with stories about benefits of being 'circumcised'? By using force to reach her genitalia, knifing her vulva, tying her legs, isolating her, forbidding her to wash, discouraging her from schooling, or marrying her young? I don't think so.

FGM is, we can agree, contrary to the interests of the child. Telling her it's good teaches her to lie; heaping gifts on her teaches her corruption; bullying her teaches meanness; hiding the risks teaches her deception. Are these the qualities that governments want in their citizens? And even if the girl child is not regarded as even potentially a voter, should the interests of the parents, who act on economic motives, trump the child's? Not according to international conventions that Kenya has signed.

The Convention inspires action to put legal and administrative measures in place that obviate against these violations. Parental authority should be limited, at least where decisions to amputate a clitoris and marry off a daughter are concerned. Medical facilities should be provided – constructed if needed – and adequately staffed. Government should ensure that institutions, facilities and services for care and protection of children exist and that all should conform to professional standards.

In addition to educational and health entitlements, the CRC guarantees certain privileges of citizenship. Performing FGM without the girl's consent, for instance, breaches children's right to form and express their own opinions, as stipulated in Article 12 (1). Their views are invited in "all matters affecting them," and, according to the child's maturity and age, her thoughts should be given weight. ACRWC Article 7, moreover, on Freedom of Expression, reinforces the importance of this right.

Let's reiterate a key phrase here bracketing the child's "maturity and age." This implies that even if the child, aware of FGM, does not rebel, she is often too young to understand or give informed consent. She may also be responding to the threat of exclusion. Possibly mocked by age-mates, she chooses what seems to be the lesser evil. More often, though, she isn't consulted at all.

National instruments for child protection in Kenya

In line with obligations accepted as a signatory to the United Nation's Human Rights and Children's Rights Conventions and the ACRWC, Kenya passed the Children's Act in 2011.

This Act of Parliament makes provision for parental responsibility, fostering, adoption, custody, maintenance, guardianship, care and protection of children. It also makes provision for the administration of children's institutions, gives effect to the principles of the Convention on the Rights of the Child and the African Charter on the Rights and Welfare of the Child.[5]

Paragraphs relevant to female genital mutilation see it as a violation of the rights of the child and include sections 14 (1) – "No person shall subject a child to female circumcision, early marriage or other cultural rites, customs or traditional practices that are likely to negatively affect the child's life, health, social welfare, dignity or physical or psychological development" [ibid] – and 119 (h) which further provides that a child in need of care and protection is a female subjected to or threatened with undergoing "female circumcision" or early marriage. Additional customs or practices "detrimental to the life, education and health of the child" are similarly proscribed.

I welcome this legislative gesture for it clearly criminalizes FGM (and the booking of young girls for marriage, intimately tied to its prerequisite, the cutting). This progressive effort notwithstanding, and despite the Act's enactment over a decade ago, rampant cases of abuse of children's rights, namely FGM, continue almost unabated, as reported regularly from various parts of the country. Despite the weakening hold of traditional culture and other dynamics of modernization, FGM is stubborn and the Children's Act is gathering dust. It hasn't been applied.

Why not?

Community leaders in affected districts, mainly pastoral groups, maintain that FGM is a cultural practice, an important rite of passage, and a necessary prerequisite for marriage – as we have seen. They insist on its utility in preserving 'purity', a bias against the female sex. Furthermore, they resent the federal government encroachment on their local political prerogative. They strongly believe that legislating customs – for or against – is their responsibility and theirs alone. Aware of the federal law and the sanctions imposed for violation, they nonetheless discount the distant power and stipulate the legitimacy of their own. Indeed, whenever culture clashes with law, communities privilege home rule and accept the threat of prosecution and imprisonment to protect their traditional way of life.

This impunity has been perpetuated by a system of inefficient law enforcement whose employees, for the most part, had not participated in the formulation of the Act. Local administrators, expected to raise the alarm when the Act is breached, give allegiance first to their culture and only secondarily to their profession. After all, police officers are part of the community and more than likely think like the majority. In any case, from their perspective, standing against the procedure would be betraying their culture and their peers. They therefore strongly believe that elders and councils of elders should deal with cultural concerns, not the courts. In some instances, interference and threats by chiefs and councilors against those who rescue girls running away from FGM have been reported. Still, harmonizing culture and law is crucial, especially for uncut girls who do indeed have trouble finding spouses. As do migrants: to avoid losing potential local suitors for their daughters, families in Maasai territory who have come from non-'circumcising' groups find themselves pushed to embrace the cut.

Moreover, religious beliefs have hindered full implementation of the Act, especially in Muslim zones. The erroneous conviction that FGM is Islamic has led some to discount the decree. After all, doesn't God's law trump human ones? Advocates of this view call FGM "Sunna," believe it is acceptable and deny claims of excessive pain. And the possibility remains that they may not understand the law. Opinion leaders may have trouble with its technicality, and it may be inaccessible in local languages, thus posing further challenges to implementation.

I welcome Kenya's Children's Act, as noted before, but I recognize one, hopefully temporary, drawback. Cutting communities, going to great lengths to escape the reaches of the law, have taken the practice underground. This, too, has already been shown, but not in the context of hope that legal sanctions augured a fairly rapid end to FGM. Privatization among the Maasai points in the opposite direction. What had been performed in the open has simply gone indoors and is now arranged privately by households. Similarly, a minor shift toward medicalization shields perpetrators from the law. A diagnosis can be made; an anesthetic administered; an amputation managed; and the healing hidden. If a clinical setting offers some reprieve to the girl on the operating table, mainly anesthesia (and here I won't impugn the advantage of this to the victim), FGM remains a travesty of the child's body, and medicalization universally condemned by most activists for women's dignity.

Another result of the changes in venue is increased impenetrability and difficulty in bringing clinicians and parents to justice. One thing is clear, though: performed now at almost any age in childhood, and in the absence of communal celebration, – public rituals are dying out –, the naked truth of the custom's aim stands out. Not a 'rite of passage', it sets the clock for women back. Not empowering for the girl under the knife, it does the opposite – disables her.

And the punishment? The Act reads, Article 20:

Notwithstanding penalties contained in any other law, where any person willfully or as a consequence of culpable negligence infringes any of the rights of a child as specified in sections 5 to 19, such person shall be liable upon summary conviction to a term of imprisonment not exceeding twelve months, or to a fine not exceeding fifty thousand shillings or to both such imprisonment and fine.[6]

Seemingly clear on what awaits abusers of girls' clitorises, in fact the Children's Act in Kenya leaves it to the prudence of the magistrates to determine sentencing for FGM. No specific penalties for this violation appear.

What do I suggest we do to reinforce human rights of the girl child?

I've taken the time to describe these international conventions because Kenya is party to them, and it seems to me, working through and with them, insisting that they be upheld, is the best way to go. And since Kenya as a member state adopted the CRC and ACRWC and integrated them into the Children's Act of 2001, our focus should shift towards implementing the Children's Act.

The importance of law enforcement notwithstanding, applying the law would have been far more successful had cultural concerns not been at the forefront in affected communities.

But they are, and this fact, in my view, means other approaches are also needed. Supplementing sensitization and advocacy, behavior change models can be brought in, too. In the instances where community stakeholders come together and conspire against specific government legislation, one key question is: why do they conspire against the Children's Act? This is evident in the fact that the

Children's Act, especially sections 14 and 119 (1) (h), has simply not been enforced. Those mandated to apply it seem inadequately prepared to do so, especially local administrators at grass roots level whose allegiance, as we have seen, is not to a central government edict but to their own municipality.

Despite most stakeholders' awareness of provisions in the Children's Act, it's discouraging to realize that so far, this knowledge has not been translated into definitive or action-oriented mechanisms. Furthermore, police and the courts, key actors in implementing the law, are underutilized; they handle very few cases, if any at all. Nor has local government been cooperative in moving forward against FGM.

A rights-based analysis and approach to abandonment is therefore an effective solution to the loud outcry of cut girls like me. Specific groups to target include parents, government (administration) officers, young girls, i.e. children, community leaders or elders and faith-based organizations or FBOs, together with Non-Governmental Organizations (NGOs), Civil Society Organizations and Community-based Organizations (CBO's). A lasting solution presupposes joint effort.

Ideally, what I would like to see is an umbrella association, one through which all stakeholders might have a say and which, basing its recommendations on objective data, could approach the issue from two broad perspectives, initially looking at government's potential duties and then focusing on cutting communities and their information needs.

I recommend interrogating government's role in ending FGM by reviewing the Children's Act of 2001 to seal loopholes in theory and examine hindrances to application. Gaps in the Children's Act that the umbrella group working with government might address include the following.

First, a consultative review of the Children's Act would reveal the lack of relevant stakeholder involvement. Where were the councils of elders, community leaders, parents and CBOs at the community level when sections 14 (I) and 119 (h) were discussed? To create sustainable ownership of the process, input on FGM must be sought and considered.

Second, the Act itself is a long and comprehensive document. Government should provide unambiguous rules for implementing clauses in the Act against FGM.

Third, the umbrella committee and government should themselves be clear about the non-admissibility of any form of community dispute resolution in cases of FGM. We really shouldn't let the fox guard the hens! Adjudication should remain the sole responsibility of the courts, thereby taking FGM out of the hands of the council of elders.

Fourth, government should develop specific protocols to train and monitor provincial administrators, enabling them to implement the Children's Act at community level. Training should also consider how best to select local employees who do not feel owned by their culture.

Fifth, government must ensure that the Act is made widely available and that a protocol is in place concerning dissemination. The Act must be written in simple language and be reader friendly, even to people with minimal education like the village elders. The reviewed Act should be translated into native languages for people at the grassroots to understand.

Sixth, government should make provisions for minimum sentencing and penalties for FGM-related offences and also empower Children's Officers to initiate and prosecute FGM-relevant cases.

Seventh, government should be mobilized to ensure that FGM is integrated into the curriculum, especially in primary schools. This would strongly contribute to young girls' awareness of negative impacts and counter-act enticement by parents and elders who hide the truth behind claims that it's 'good'.

Eighth, media should be brought in to increase cognizance of FGM using local stations, indigenous languages and presenters from the region. This will help to reach more people and especially those who may not access regular meetings.

Ninth, partnerships should be encouraged, linking CBOs and government to scale up the process of monitoring anti-FGM activities at the grassroots level. Political leaders, ex-circumcisers, councils of elders, FBOs, youth, *morans* (warriors) and like-minded stakeholders in anti-FGM advocacy can pair off to cooperate effectively.

Tenth, opinion leaders and influential committees at community level should be trained to support implementation of the Act and monitor FGM activities.

Eleventh, government in partnership with the umbrella group or its constituent associations should scale up technical, legal and financial support to non-profits already working on FGM at community level, thereby enhancing their impact.

Twelfth, government should be assisted to develop community-friendly Information Education and Communication materials, both audio and visual, on anti-FGM advocacy.

My second broad approach, looking at communities for their information needs, is clearly as crucial as government engagement. For now the question is concretely, what might persuade the cutting groups to stop? I have the following suggestions.

First, help local agencies already present shift their focus towards hosting rescue camps for girls who run away from home during 'circumcision' season and aim to develop a broader shelter network. A clearly identified, locally acceptable Alternative Rite of Passage (ARP) might also be encouraged to abandon cutting without sacrificing the appeal of pageantry. The Rescue Camps should be prepared to teach others to advocate against FGM and try an ARP ceremony. An intensive community sensitization program combined with a public ARP celebration fully integrated into a girls' empowerment platform can be effective in encouraging abandonment.

Second, cooperate with local NGOs and civil servants to persuade the Maasai Council of Elders and other opinion-leaders to become agents of change against FGM. The influence they exert on the lives of the Maasai people makes them key players, and their conversion can spell failure or success for campaigns. Currently, fear of repercussions in going against the wishes of the Council is perhaps the prime social pressure maintaining the practice. Indeed, these elders have the power to declare that families whose girls remain uncut shall be considered outcasts.

Third, develop interventions that focus on empowerment to help girls cope with the stress,– peer pressure and bullying--, intended to force them to submit to FGM. For instance, extra-curricular clubs in schools could teach life-skills while offering information and training to resist both family insistence and classmates' hazing. More ARP programs could extend activities as well.

Fourth, increase community education focusing on the negative health and social effects of FGM including its illegality. Address all community members in a local language that can be easily understood. Programs should engage everyone in pedagogy in the broadest sense: staff, teachers, village and church leaders, traditional circumcisers and health professionals.

Fifth, enlist government and local agencies to strengthen public awareness of existing laws forbidding FGM and ensure the process of reporting cases to the authorities is known. You can also, in addition, push local government to enforce the law with increased diligence.

Sixth, partner with local agencies to build upon initiatives identified as promising in the fight to stop FGM, such as encouraging girls to stay in school, supporting teachers who discuss FGM in mixed groups, urging churches to actively oppose it, or implementing girls' empowerment and ARP programs. Don't forget the more marginalized members of the community, in particular those families outside the school networks, many of whom have limited levels of literacy.

Seventh, merge with local agencies to engage men and community leaders in initiatives to abandon FGM. Although the practice is seen as largely a women's affair, men have a role to play as heads of households providing resources for the celebration. The community needs to be persuaded that cultures can and do change, and it is not necessary to cling to a practice whose purpose is upholding cultural tradition.

Eighth, with local agencies, engage the community in discussion of sexual morality and FGM, conveying your view that ethical behavior is not coerced by amputation but promoted by education, and if once a stated aim of FGM had been to ensure chastity, sexual activity among young people is a societal issue not solved by cutting. Words are more eloquent than knives.

Ninth, assist government to oppose involvement of medical staff in perpetuating FGM. Less leniency toward violators is needed. In the past, the Ministry of Health has implicitly forbidden medicalization with a general prohibition, but it appears not to have succeeded in changing behaviour. It is important to revisit this issue and enforce the law more effectively with stricter sanctions which may be reviewed to include withdrawal of offending clinicians' licenses.

Tenth, schools provide an excellent avenue for addressing FGM and encouraging youth to reject it, yet teachers feel inhibited because, after all, it has something to do with sex and sex is, throughout the world, an intergenerational challenge. To remedy this, I recommend partnering with teacher training institutions helping faculty overcome social inhibitions and enabling them to address FGM in class.

Eleventh, support government's efforts to strengthen enforcement of existing laws prohibiting FGM and promoting children's rights. As we have seen, community leaders know FGM is illegal but deliberately choose to flout the law. Explicit protocols are therefore needed to guide reporting, investigating and prosecuting offenders. Results must also be monitored and made known.

Finally, merge with local agencies and partners to build successful strategies that lead to rejection of FGM among the Maasai. For instance, the church has significant influence. Working more closely with religious institutions might improve the reach and sustainability of abandonment programs.

Notes

1 To learn more about the Inter African Committee, visit http://www.iac-ciaf.net/ where you will find the history, a declaration of principles and, at present, eulogies for four leaders who recently passed away, including Efua Dorkenoo OBE. Website retrieved 11 May 2015.

2 "Article 15 - Freedom from torture or cruel, inhuman or degrading treatment or punishment." United Nations Enable. Development and Human Rights for All. http://www.un.org/disabilities/default.asp?id=275. Retrieved 8 October 2014.

3 http://daccess-dds-ny.un.org/doc/RESOLUTION/GEN/NR0/043/88/IMG/NR004388. pdf?OpenElement Retrieved 20 July 2014.

4 Ibid.

5 http://www.chr.up.ac.za/undp/domestic/docs/legislation_03.pdf Retrieved 20 July 2014.

6 http://www.chr.up.ac.za/undp/domestic/docs/legislation_03.pdf Retrieved 20 July 2014.

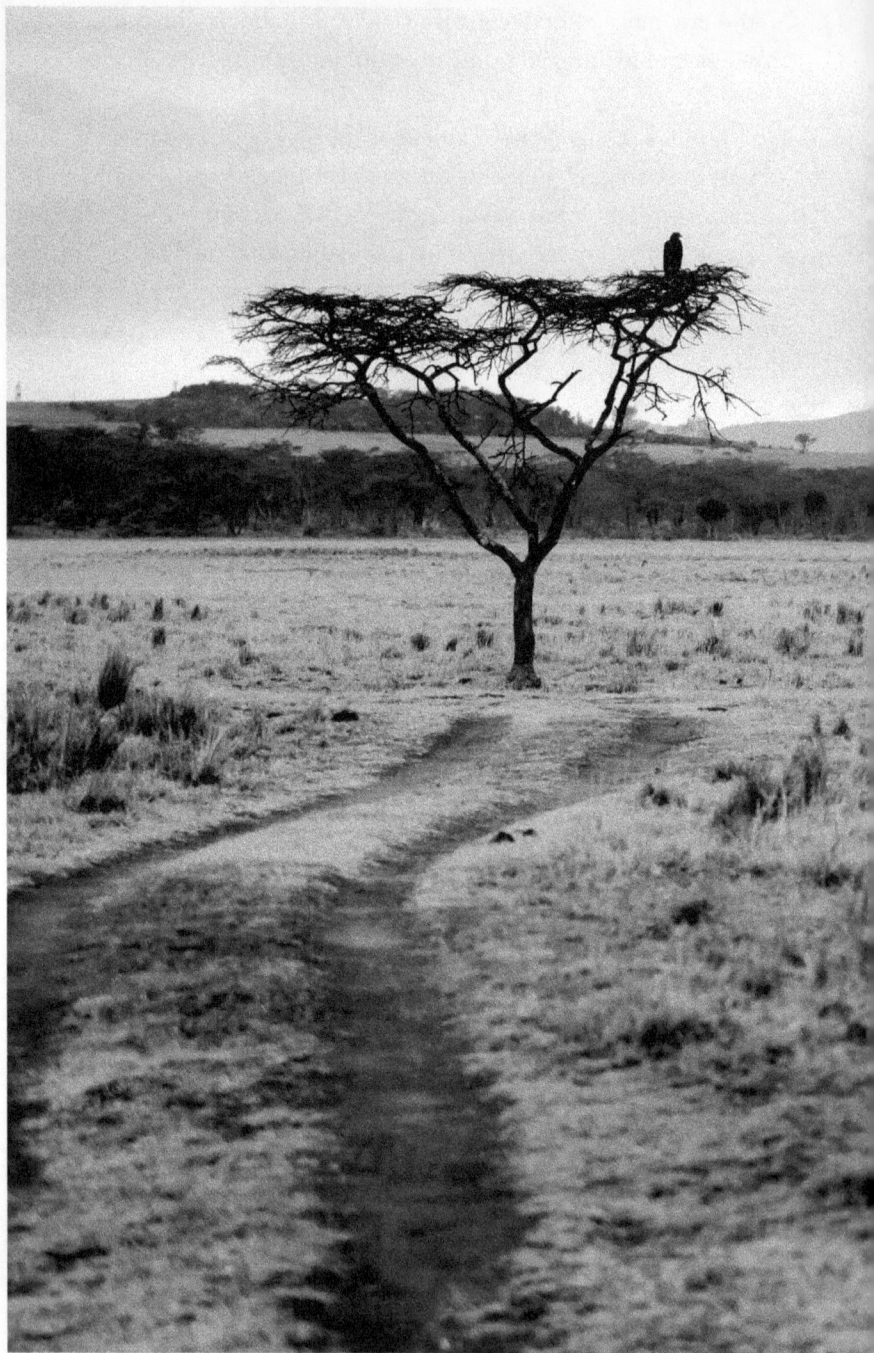

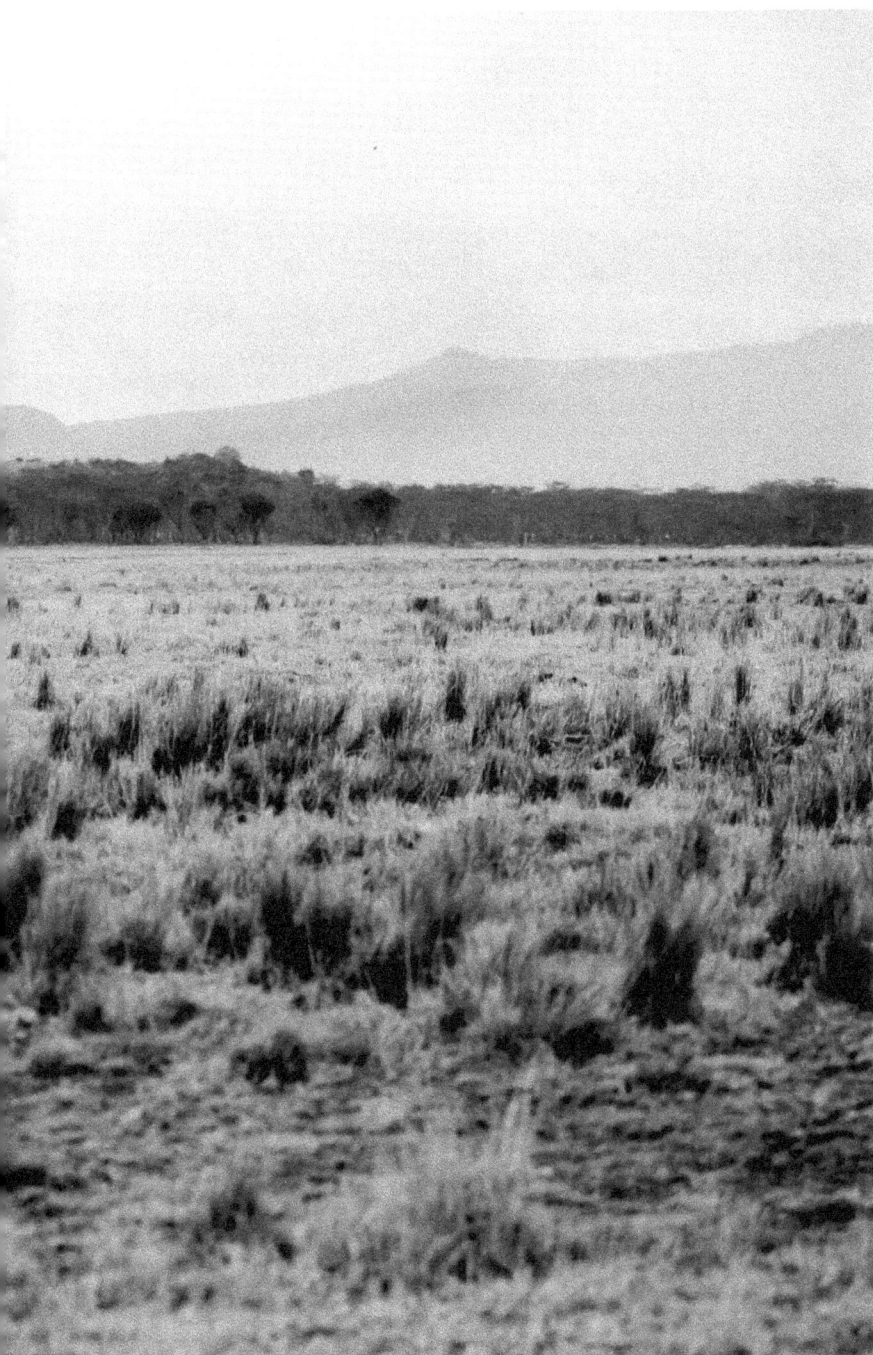

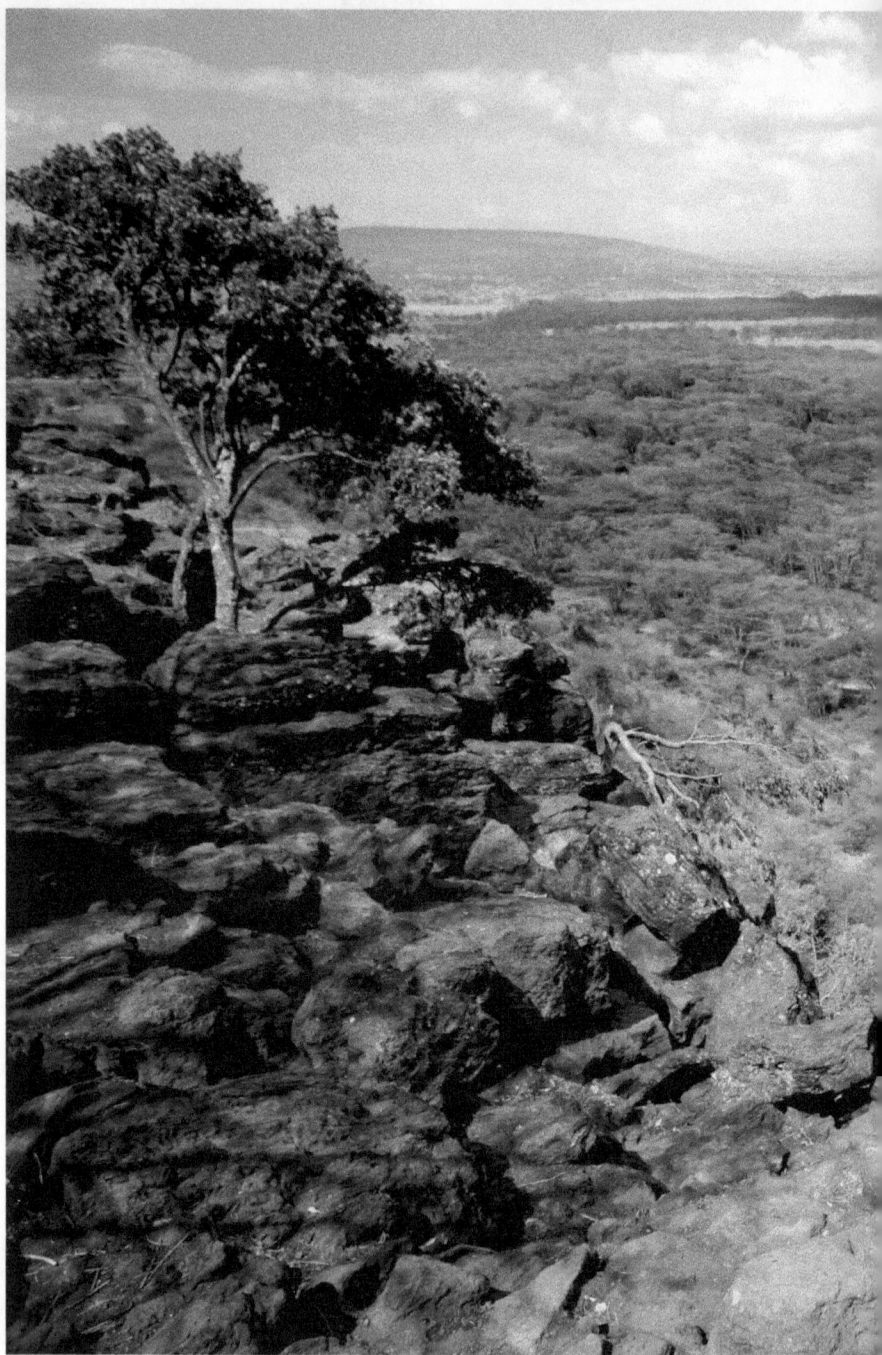

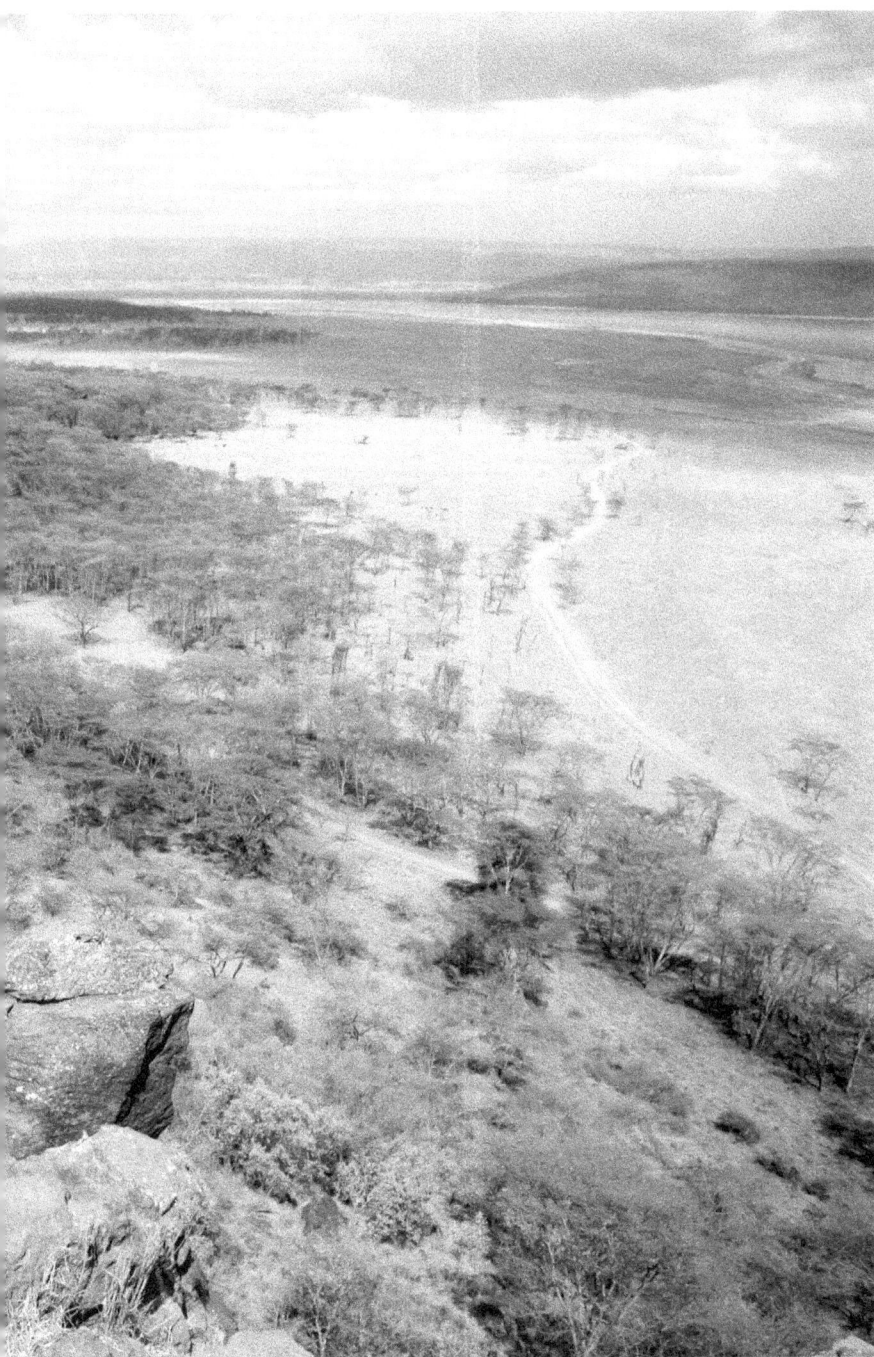

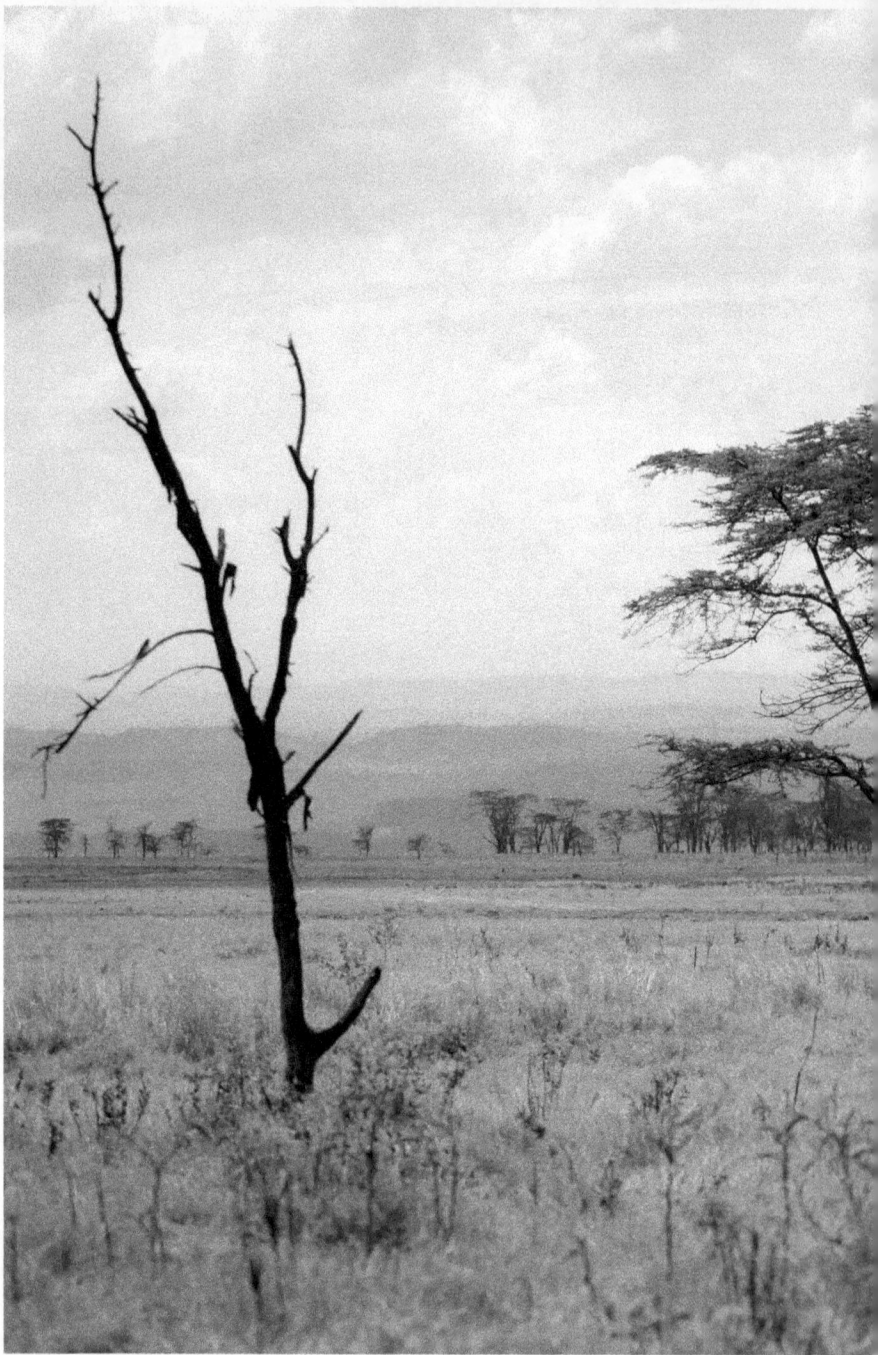

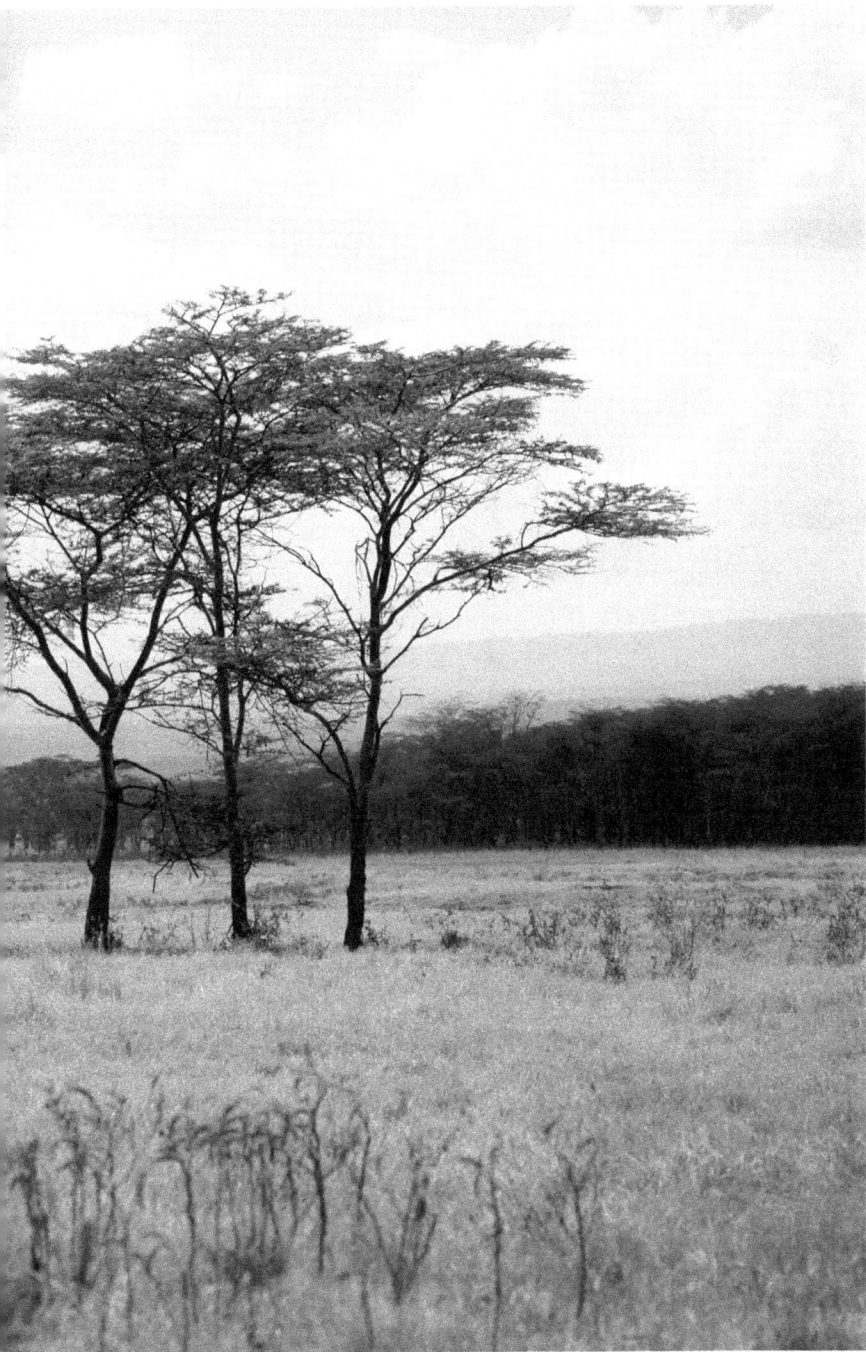

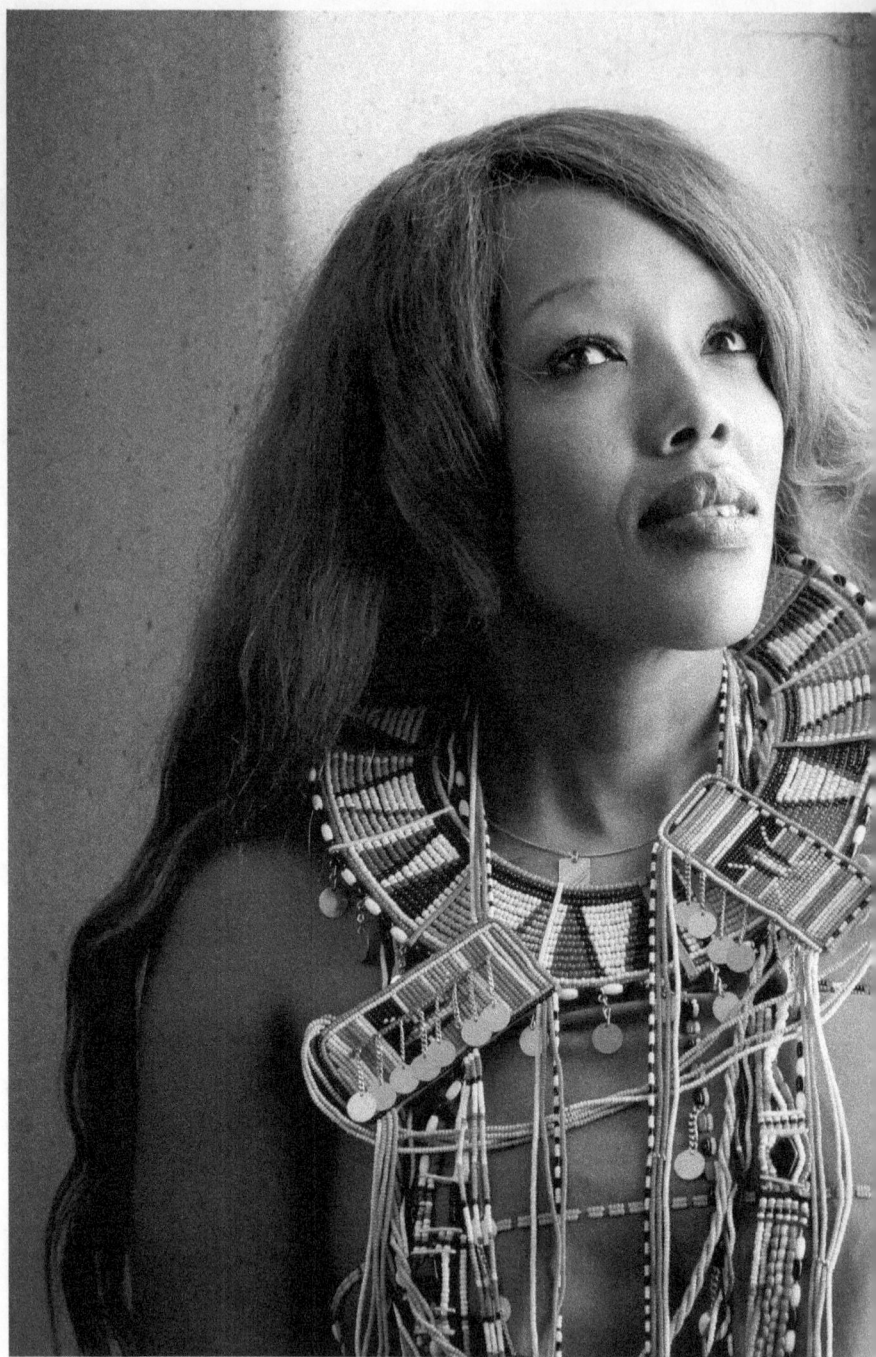

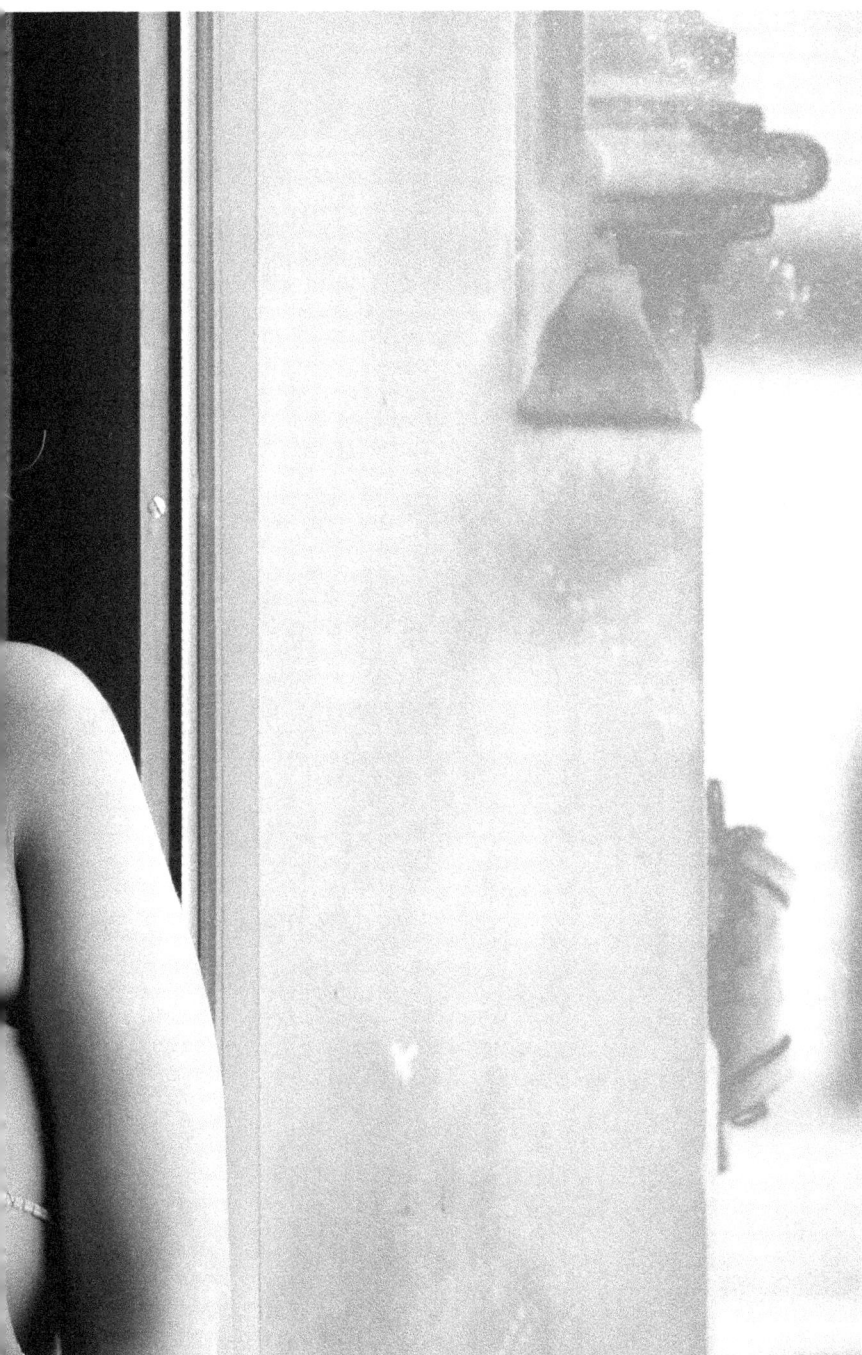

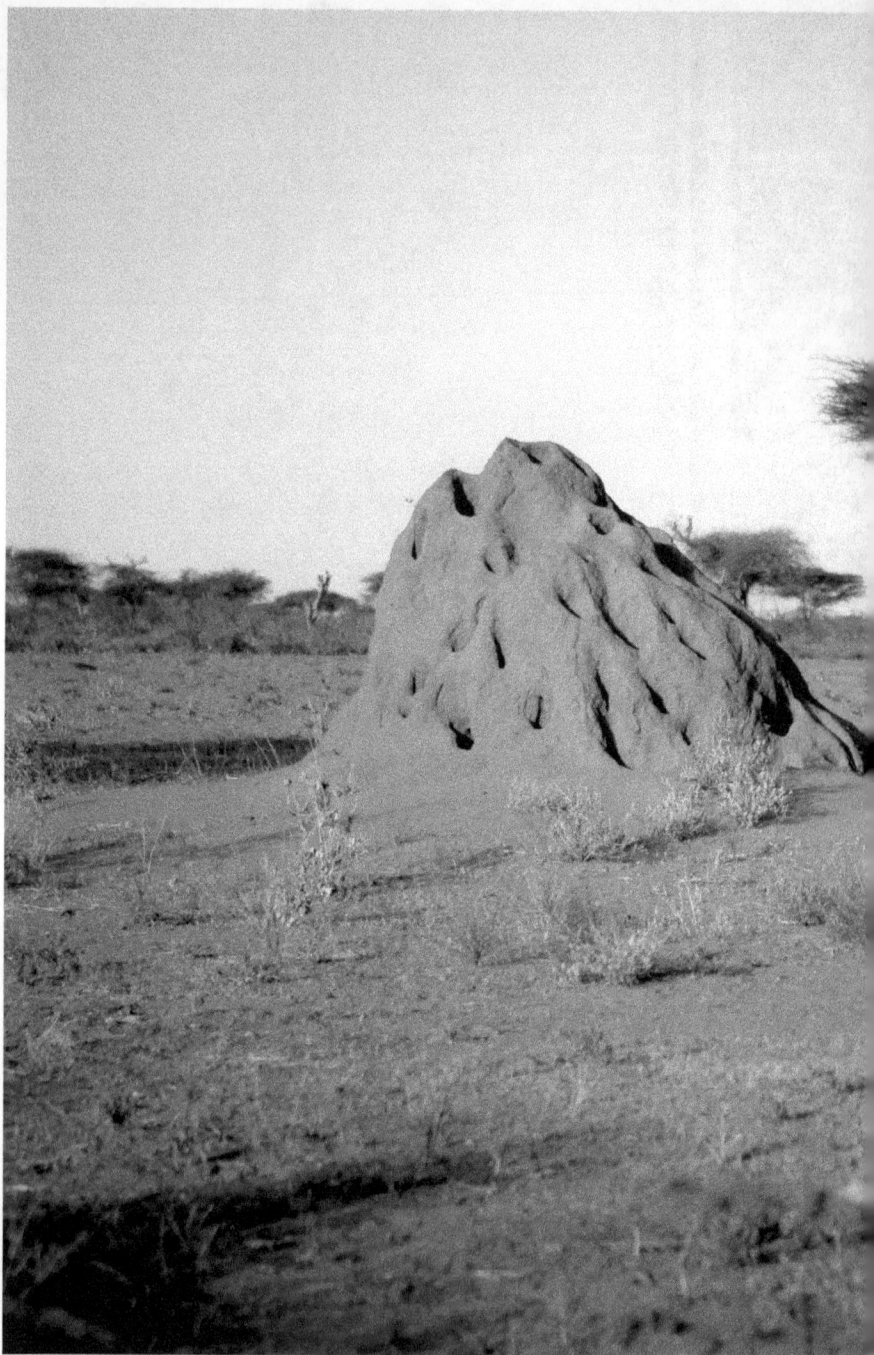

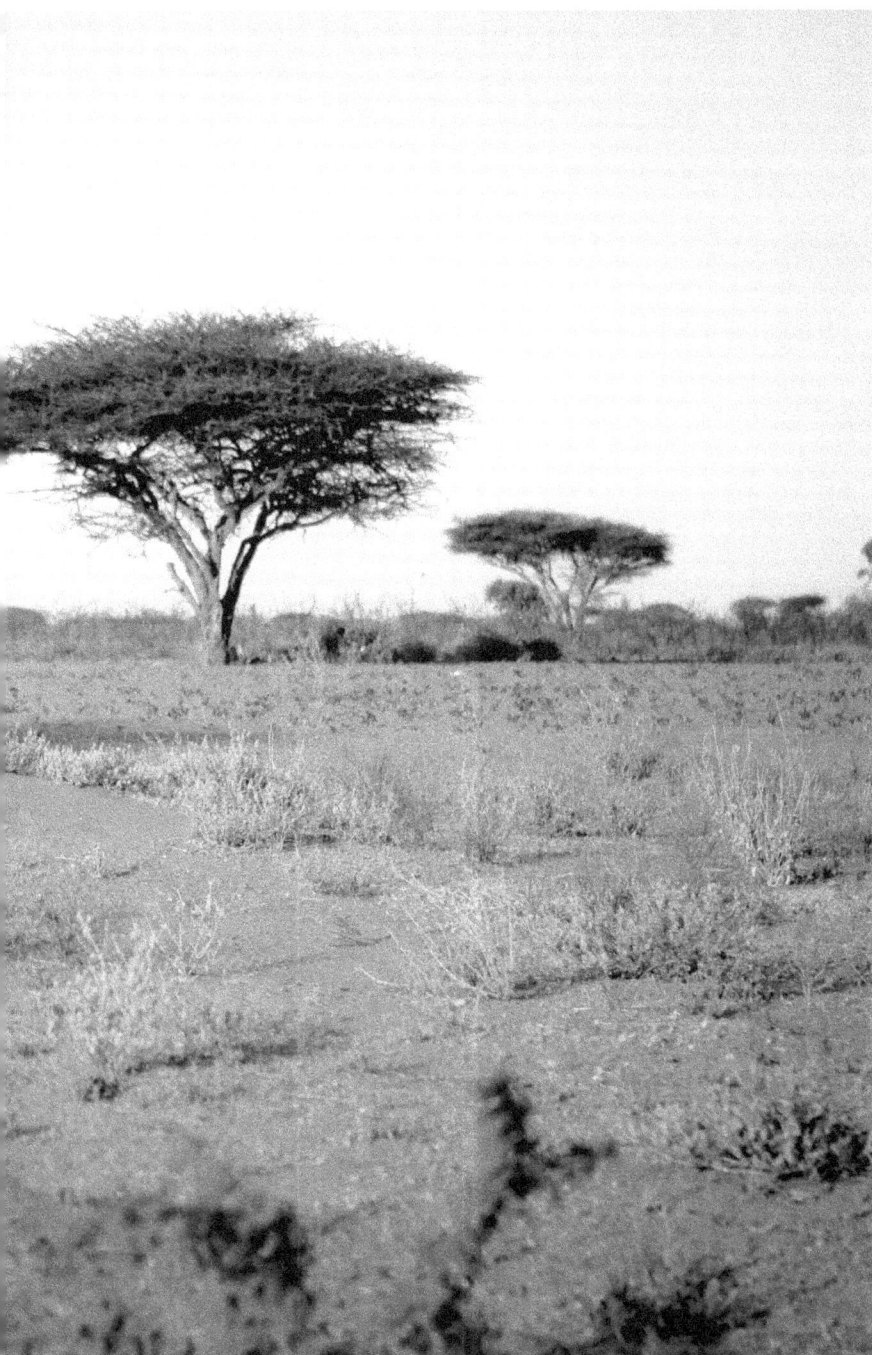

THE SOURCEBOOK

Myths of the Maasai: FGM Engagement, Postcolonial Lens

Noel Ciqi Duan

Given heavy media coverage of FGM that will often exoticize and 'other' the Maasai, Maria Kiminta, a member of the tribe, portrays the cut as she endured it. Speaking out not only as an activist but also as a role model for young girls growing up in similar circumstances, she encourages resistance from within.

The Maasai, although connected by the Maa language, are actually comprised of many different groups that inhabit the African Great Lakes region. As anthropologist Dorothy Hodgson explains in her ethnography, *Once Intrepid Warriors: Gender, Ethnicity, and the Cultural Politics of Maasai Development,* individuals who currently count as Maasai did not originally consider themselves one people. The very idea of an "indigenous" folk emerged from postcolonial globalization in order to mobilize social and political action—such as the fight against FGM, and conversely, the fight *for* FGM, as well.

One of the most poignant moments in Maria's memoir occurs at the beginning when she describes the misinformation that sisters, other relatives and friends give about the process itself. She asks, "[W]ho wouldn't want to enjoy the elevated social status that came with [FGM]?" The betrayal and lies – from older girls ostracizing younger girls to not being allowed near the "circumcision" room – reflect a desire to protect custom and "indigenous" practices. Now, Maria argues that she is not per se against traditional ways. "I would like to see the Maasai community conserve their rich culture," she writes, "retaining ceremonial rituals such as feasting and blessings on initiates, but in the absence of amputating women's sexual organs." You find in much anthropological theory an appreciation of how local culture can provide insight – and inject tension – into the global community. Maria's story is her unique tale, but it reflects and challenges our own biases, presuppositions, and beliefs.

Additionally, as an anthropologist, I choose not to intervene with the subjects of study, aiming for transparency in self-reflexive research – but as a women's studies student and feminist activist, the line of so-called objectivity remains elusive when dealing with certain ethical issues. I'm not convinced that objectivity, raised to a pedestal by male Enlightenment thinkers, is equally suited to all disciplines – especially when they deal with FGM. Because women's studies scholars relate so personally to their work and so much of feminist scholarship comes from political motivation – more so, say, than your typical economist dealing with sharp graphs of supply and demand – it feels impossible to be immersed in women's studies and *not* become an activist! Emotion, associated with femaleness and for that reason degraded as less valuable an epistemology than rationality and distance, is an integral aspect of both motivation-driven research and activism. After all, motivation-driven research thrives not on the lack of involvement that an emphasis on *ratio* demands but on emotion, and if passion has typically been linked to the female to shame her, it lies in our power to revive subjectivity when it comes to a topic as ethically-challenging as FGM.

So, Maria aptly calls her script *Speaking Out against FGM*, bravely – and contentiously – challenging readers not to separate the emotional and personal from public policies and scholarly research. The protagonist asks us to suspend our biases against external intervention as detrimental to the Maasai way of life and to abandon our indifference toward – and thus implied approval of – "indigenous" practices in general. While Western feminists are often criticized for intervening on behalf of – that is, "saving" – non-white women, the objection is hardly applicable here, as Maria is speaking out as an FGM survivor herself and a Maasai. Detailing her experience in all its horror, she is clear about the need for res-cue, not by outside 'whites' but by the government of Kenya, called on to pass laws and apply them.

Maria Kiminta's passion notwithstanding, it will take much more than a memoir, however good, to wipe out FGM. Patience, education and time are essential. Nonetheless, activist research is not an oxymoron; activism and scholarship can enhance one another in a mutually beneficial symbiosis.

What Maria does successfully is to de-exoticize her people, the Maasai, who are often seen as a tribe romantically maintaining their pastoral ways amidst growing capitalist pressures. Although like any other "nationality," they have been shaped by history, par-ticularly colonial history, Maria doesn't mystify her group's prac-tices and beliefs. Instead, she describes the hard truth of FGM, including deception and dishonesty vis-à-vis excision candidates, yet showing that in spite of this and the pain it brings, she respects the power of the elders and upholds beneficial traditions.

This task is all the more important given the Maasai's formative role in the Western world's perception of Africa – they appear, seemingly ubiquitous, wearing their tribal garments, colorful beads and Shúkà (sheets wrapped around the body) in tourism pamph-lets, magazines, movies, airline advertisements, and other forms of communication. In these popular media, however, while digni-fied, they also seem "primitive" and frozen in time as the *bon sauv-age*, or noble savage, childlike in innocence and uncorrupted by civilization – a regrettable distortion.

As noted by D.L. Hodgson in *Once Intrepid Warriors*,[1] the Maa-speaking peoples were originally agro-pastoralists in areas now known as Tanzania and Kenya. However, enabled by mastery of iron forging, decades of high rainfall, and social organization, some groups of Maa-speakers became pure pastoralists, a process consolidated under British colonization of the area in the 1800s when Maasai "reserves" were created to contain these previously semi-nomadic Maa-speaking tribes. As Hodgson discovers, women's disenfranchisement within the Maasai community emerged largely out of colonial development. As Homewood, Coast and Thompson confirm: "Current work suggests women played an active part in management and decision-making, but that from the advent of the colonial period, they were progressively excluded from rights over land, livestock and resource management and became juridical minors and dependents (Hodgson 2000)."[2]

Historical documents show how the British Empire, in order to increase rates of livestock production, encouraged the marginaliza-tion and isolation of the Maasai through the Maasai Reserve and other development implementations. Women were encouraged to be subjugated to Maasai men, as pastoralist property became as-sociated with an increasingly brittle masculine identity. Maa-sai men, under the yoke of the British, felt emasculated under the colonists' control. Recent activities initiated by the Nigerian and Tanzanian governments – such as conservation acts – and develop-ment NGOs have only strengthened the linkage of pastoralism and Maasai masculine identity.

Thus, it becomes clear that examining postcolonial gender rela-tions is essential to understanding Maria's account of FGM. Al-though an accusatory finger is pointed at a custom that has prov-en so cruel in the protagonist's own life and has devastated many others' fates, Maria's underlying empathy for elders who excise girls acknowledges the last few centuries' complex historical and social processes to which perpetrators have been exposed. After all, where the social fabric is so tightly woven, no single individual can be held accountable for FGM's tenacity and longevity. Maria makes clear that governments are responsible for protecting child-ren – this isn't simply a domestic question. In fact, it is partly be-cause FGM is considered a private family decision that it has been extremely controversial and difficult to eradicate. Maria pushes for making FGM a public issue of child welfare, elevating the subject to one of national and international concern. Speaking out, she testifies against the silence that has shrouded FGM for much too long and offers hope that bringing it out in the open can help to end it.

References

1 Hodgson, D.L. 2001. *Once intrepid warriors: gender, ethnicity, and the cultural politics of Maasai development.* Bloomington: Indiana University Press.
2 Homewood, K. and Coast, Ernestina and Thompson, D. M. (2004) "In-migrants and exclusion in east African rangelands: access, tenure and conflict." *Africa*, 74 (4). pp. 567-610. Here p. 569. ISSN 0001-9720. DOI: 10.3366/afr.2004.74.4.567 © 2004 Cambridge University Press

This version available at: http://eprints.lse.ac.uk/270/

In LSE Research Online: August 2012. Retrieved 10 June 2015.

FGM Amongst the Maasai of Kenya

Equality Now, Nairobi[1]

The following appeared as chapters two and three in *Protecting Girls from Undergoing Female Genital Mutilation. The Experience of Working with Maasai Communities in Kenya and Tanzania*, a booklet published by Equality Now in cooperation with NAFGEM and TASARU Girls' Rescue Center, originally adapted from the article "In-depth: Razor's Edge - The Controversy of Female Genital Mutilation. FGM among the Maasai Community in Kenya" in *IRIN News*, the humanitarian news and analysis service of the UN Office for the Coordination of Humanitarian Affairs, Nairobi, 1 March 2005 (IRIN INDEPTH). Available from <www.irinnews.org> Booklet first published 2011 by Equality Now <http:/www.equalitynow.org>

A semi-nomadic community located in several districts of central Kenya and northern Tanzania, the Maasai wander in search of pasture and water for their animals. The population has been estimated at about 1 million in both Kenya and Tanzania but the figure is likely to be inaccurate, given the group's erstwhile reluctance to cooperate with government census-takers.[2]

Although both Kenya and Tanzania have encouraged the Maasai to abandon their semi-nomadic lifestyle, they remain a proud people who have famously retained distinctive customs, culture and dress in spite of pressure to conform to modernization and Western influence.

Traditionally, cow's milk, maize meal and meat have fulfilled the tribe's need for nourishment (although meat consumption has decreased). The Maasai grow or rear all of this food, reducing their need to rely on other communities, which has in turn limited their exposure to and influence from other nations.

Given this ingrained sense of culture and tradition, persuading the Maasai to abandon customary practices like FGM faces a considerable challenge.

The Origin of FGM amongst the Maasai

According to Maasai myth, a girl called Napei once had inter-course with an enemy of her family. To punish her and suppress the desires that lead her to commit such a crime, Napei was sub-jected to female genital mutilation. Since then, nearly every female Maasai adolescent has undergone FGM, used to curb female sexual desire and promiscuity. Conversely, girls who face the blade bring honor to themselves and their families.

As a result, despite massive domestic and international criticism, the Maasai have held on to the custom. Criminalization of FGM in Kenyan law in 2001 has also had little effect. Even educated men and women, aware of the risks, continue excision for fear of rejec-tion by wider Maasai society. For regardless of how educated she may be or how high her social status, an 'uncircumcised' Maasai woman is considered and treated like a child and risks isolation from the community as well as zero-to-nil prospects of finding a Maasai spouse.

The FGM ceremony

The Maasai ceremony is a large annual community celebration for all girls who have reached adolescence during the year. Festiv-ities feature groups mostly between 12 and 14 who undergo FGM on the same day; they are cut by traditional 'circumcisers' (usually ex-perienced elderly women). Until recently, the same sharp instru-ment (often a fine-bladed knife known as an "ormurunya") maimed all the candidates; now, under threat of HIV, different tools are used.

After cutting and to stop bleeding, a paste made from cow dung and milk fat is applied to the wound.

Clitoridectomy, the type of FGM most common among the Maasai, involves the removal of the visible part of the clitoris.[3] Its physical effects include:

° severe pain (performed without anesthetics)
° bleeding (at times lethal)
° infection (especially due to poor sanitary conditions)
° complications during childbirth (often leading to stillbirths)
° keloid scarring and cysts formation and
° reduced sexual sensation

After undergoing FGM, the girls enter seclusion to be taught females' rights and duties. Once returned to the village, they are considered fully grown, marriageable women. FGM is thus tied into the community's sense of honor.

Changing the Maasai Position on FGM

In spite of their ingrained sense of culture and tradition, the Maasai have shown a degree of openness to change. ...

For example, use of the same knife on several girls has dropped in popularity to only 14% (according to studies by the NGO, Maendeleo Ya Wanawake [MYWO] in Kenya). This reduction has been attributed to increased community awareness of the role played by shared knives and the potential to transmit diseases like HIV/AIDS.

Alternative rites-of-passage (ARP) also discourage FGM. Blades have no place in such rituals. Their intact genitals notwithstanding, initiates are taught their roles as women as well as offered lessons on sexual and reproductive health and the importance of formal education.

However, the extent to which men will be prepared to pay the bride price for girls who have enjoyed alternative rites and graduated with the clitoris intact is unknown.

Although FGM is against Kenyan law, neither Maasai excisers nor parents face probable prosecution or other repercussions. Despite globalization, the Maasai remain singularly proud of their history, practices, and culture, so that anyone seeking to alter those norms – including FGM – faces an uphill task.

Nonetheless, hope exists. The Maasai are open to change on their own terms. Increasing numbers of pupils are enrolling in formal educational institutions. There, the youngsters are likely to learn about the risks associated with FGM and cultivate attitudes favorable to abandonment.

FGM CASE STUDY FROM THE MAASAI COMMUNITY IN THE NAROK DISTRICT, KENYA

According to the 2008/9 Kenya Demographic and Health Surveys (KDHS), the national prevalence of FGM amongst women between 15 and 49 is 27%.[4] This aggregate data, however, hides the differences among ethnic groups. Numbers are far higher among the Somali (98%), Kisii (96%), and the Maasai (73%) while figures remain relatively low among the Kikuyu, Kamba and Turkana, and shrink even further among the Luo and Luhya (less than 1%).[5]

FGM incidence therefore varies tremendously by province, ranging from 1% in Western province to 98% in North Eastern province. Roughly one-third of women in Eastern, Nyanza, and Rift Valley provinces have undergone FGM compared with over a quarter in the Central province. 14% of those are in Nairobi and 10 % in Coast province. The most severe form predominates in North Eastern province.

Overall the last decade has witnessed a decrease in national prevalence. In 2008/9, 27% of women had suffered FGM, a decline from
32% in 2003 and 38% in 1998. Moreover, the younger generation is
less likely to have been cut than the older.

The Tasaru Ntomonok Initiative (TNI)

The TNI is a Kenyan community-based organization established
in 1999 to promote awareness of women's rights and fight to end
all social and cultural practices harmful to girls and women. Based
in Narok District in the rift valley of Kenya, Tasaru Ntomonok Initiative works among the Maasai community. Agnes Pareyio, herself a
Maasai and founder/coordinator of TNI, recounts her own experience
of FGM.

Born in an ordinary Maasai village in the Enaiborr/Ajijik sub-location
of the district of Narok North, Agnes Pareyio attended Olesankale Primary School with a friend, Josephine, who came from a community
that did not practice FGM. After Josephine asked Agnes why so
many Maasai girls came back from school holidays with their hair
shaved, Agnes told her that they had been subjected to a ritual
called FGM. Josephine subsequently convinced Agnes that FGM
was wrong and advised her friend not to succumb to the practice.

In December 1965, however, Agnes went home for holidays, where
she met several people feasting. When she asked the reason for
the celebration, her mother informed her that she was going to
undergo FGM. Agnes tried to resist, seeking support from her father. Although he wanted to help, pressure from her mother, grandmother and the community proved overwhelming. It felt as though
everybody was against her.

"It ... spread in my community that I was a coward. So to prove
I'm not, I agreed to be cut," she said. The day after the amputation,

Agnes awoke in terrible pain and confusion. It took three weeks for the physical wound to heal, but long after that she continued feeling fearful, unable to trust anyone besides her father, with whom, however, she became closer as he had been the only one who tried to protect her.

After living through this horrible experience, she resolved to ensure that none of her daughters or any girls from the Maasai community would undergo what she went through. Her involvement in FGM activism started in 1984 when she began working with the national women's organization Maendeleo Ya Wanawake as a district coordinator campaigning against harmful traditional practices, including FGM.

In 1998, she encountered girls running away from the cut and realized that they urgently needed temporary housing while awaiting family reconciliation. In 2000, a group of women from V-Day in the United States provided funding to build a safe house, initially for forty-eight escapees. The refuge is now run by Tasaru Ntomonok Initiative (TNI).

TNI's Campaign against FGM

The TNI applies a multiple strategy campaign to ensure various stakeholders are reached and influenced to reject the practice. These approaches include:

(a) Community mobilization and education

Educating the Maasai community against FGM is a key feature of TNI's intervention. TNI raises community awareness through workshops and seminars that target specific groups, including community leaders (religious leaders, village chiefs, elders), 'circumcisers', teachers, women's groups, peer educators, women, men, boys and girls.

The Maasai community is male-dominated. Maasai women hold inferior positions with respect to power, decision-making and ownership of resources. As such, discussions between the sexes on FGM are rarely productive. Recognizing this, TNI holds separate seminars for women and men. This allows all participants to contribute and speak freely.

TNI Workshop with Maasai men

Both male and female groups are taught about the origin and dangers of FGM. Using IEC (information, education, communication) materials, models and films demonstrate the consequences of amputating female genitalia. Groups learn about the Children's Act of 2001, which prohibits FGM and punishes anyone who subjects a minor to it. Other crimes also find a place in the curriculum, such as rape, defilement, drug and substance abuse; sexually transmitted diseases, including HIV/AIDS, are discussed as well.

To promote deeper understanding of the dangers associated with the practice, women and girls are encouraged to share their experiences and, as a result, become increasingly empowered to say 'No' to FGM.

Moreover, TNI stresses to both the male and female groups the importance of women's education – an educated woman's earning power is significant because FGM plays a role in negotiation of bride price. Maasai men who support FGM are not infrequently motivated by economic considerations. Traditionally, FGM provides them with additional wealth through the higher amount a groom's family is willing to pay for a girl who has been cut. A girl child is therefore viewed as a source of income as soon as she is born, and fathers are becoming increasingly motivated to obtain the bride price early. This has led to reducing the age at which girls undergo FGM, some presently as young as nine being taken out of school to suffer the cut, be quickly married off and cattle received.

So, in the face of this challenging entrenchment, what has TNI been doing? The group has established community monitors to campaign against FGM, advise affected girls, and do their best to protect those at risk. This strategy, involving community members in campaigns, has given the group a sense of ownership, promoted long-term sustainability and promises more rapid erasure of the practice. Community monitors have indeed rescued and supported girls who, once taught about the horrors awaiting them if they are cut, have run away from their families to escape FGM.

(b) Protection for girls fleeing FGM

TNI provides temporary refuge to youth who flee from FGM and early marriages in the Narok South and North districts of the Rift Valley province in Kenya. It ensures that girls who have been thrown out of their homes or run away as a result of saying 'No' to FGM and/or early marriage are sheltered and supported morally, socially and educationally, and are eventually returned to their families through a reconciliatory process.

Rose Takaya (aged 13) shared her story of escaping FGM. "One day at the Full Gospel Church, I heard the pastor talk about the effect of FGM and the work of TNI. In December 2006, my father wanted to circumcise me. Although I didn't want to undergo the cut, he refused to back down, insisting that I must be circumcised. So I decided to run away to my uncle, sure he would help since he had refused to cut his daughters. But because it would have been dangerous for him if my father knew he'd had a hand in my escape, he asked his neighbor from the same church to assist. The neighbor took me to Tasaru, located approximately an hour and a half from my village. After running away, I came to learn that my younger sister had been circumcised in my place and immediately married off."

To protect girls fleeing FGM, TNI works in partnership with district authorities. Ms. Pareyio organizes workshops and seminars for local government employees, police, and teachers, whose cooperation she has gained. Once a candidate for cutting runs to the Centre or is rescued, the children's officer and police are notified. First, the children's officer ensures that the girl is safe from abuse and then applies to award legal guardianship to TNI. At the Centre, the escapees are counselled and offered even more information about the dangers of FGM.

TNI Girls' Protection Pathway

TNI's collaboration with the district children's officer and the administrative police has resulted in an informal early warning and protection mechanism that has often prevented abuse. In a number of cases, the system has not only successfully prevented FGM but has also led to the arrest and prosecution of parents and 'circumcisers' who would otherwise have gone unpunished.

Reconciliation meetings

Clearly, run-aways cannot be housed indefinitely in TNI shelters. The NGO therefore hosts reconciliation meetings between the girls and their parents.

These reunions are initially carried out between TNI, the parents and/or relatives, and the community with the help of elders and provincial administrators. In Maasai society girls are forced to undergo FGM not just by their parents, but also by others. TNI seeks to involve all stakeholders in the negotiations.

The need for extended family involvement in reconciliation emerges from the example of Dorcas, who came to the Centre to escape the cutting that her parents demanded. TNI mediated with success, the mother and father promising not to cut. Sadly, however, Dorcas and her younger sister were later forced to undergo FGM by their elder brother when their parents travelled. An inclusive approach embracing all kin and community in reconciliation helps to avoid such situations.

Reconciliation reminds parents and relatives that FGM harms health and is against the law. They are also requested to accept their daughters' decisions, to agree not to subject them to FGM or early marriage, and to permit them to continue their education. When the first get-together is successful, a second is held. Only then do the girls return home accompanied by elders and area chiefs who continue to monitor their safety; to assess their progress both at home and in school, TNI also pays regular visits. In return, beneficiaries keep in touch by letter, informing TNI in case the threat of FGM or early marriage is renewed. Because community monitors live in close proximity, girls in need are encouraged to reach out to them.

Unfortunately, not all reconciliations succeed; certain parents accept their daughters only if they agree to undergo FGM. In those cases the girls remain at the Centre for the duration of their secondary school education. Upon graduation they must leave the Centre but may choose to go back home since, as grown-up women, they are unlikely to be forcibly cut.

(c) Alternative rites of passage

Among the Maasai, as we have seen, FGM is considered a rite of passage, a sign of graduation from childhood to adulthood. During the ceremony, girls are taught to behave as women, wives, mothers, and family caretakers. That is, they are prepared for the traditional division of labor in marriage and will soon be expected to wed.

Girls at the Centre who have escaped the practice and have presumably not learned women's roles are denied recognition as women and thus face open discrimination -- being treated as children – all their lives. Hoping to alleviate this situation, TNI introduced an Alternative Rite of Passage (ARP). It offers womanhood training but eschews the cut.

The ARP instructs pupils in various topics, including Maasai culture, girl-child education, physical and sexual abuse of children, and children's human rights. Trainees are encouraged to say no to FGM and early forced marriage as well, and after five days of learning, they graduate with certificates.

This alternative rite is open not only to girls at the Centre but also to others whose parents have abandoned FGM and vowed not to mutilate their daughters. Community Monitors often identify these youth, normally between 10 and 17. Before admission, however, the youngsters must ensure fathers' and mothers' knowledge of the educational objectives and secure their agreement not to cut.

Early on, these ARP workshops faced considerable parental hostility. However, following varied and vigorous community sensitization, outreach and mobilization programs, this is changing. Girls are now allowed and at times even encouraged to undergo ARP instruction and graduate into adulthood without the cut. Instances of early marriage and FGM have thus been reduced, while female education has been promoted. The program's success has also caused boys to call for similar workshops, so that they, too, can be sensitized to the same issues and make informed, independent decisions based on their new knowledge. A good number join abolition campaigns.

(d) Promoting girls' education

TNI emphasizes the importance of girls' education and works to ensure that all housed at the Centre attend and stay in school, including run-aways who may never have been exposed to a classroom before. They receive basic instruction to smooth adaptation once they enroll.

In 2011, the Tasaru Centre in Narok hosted seventy-four escapees, forty of whom were in primary school and thirty-four in secondary. Additionally, seven girls left the Centre to pursue professional training courses and three others are now gainfully employed. Access to education and job training enables the students to provide sustainable economic and social benefits to their families and communities, thus becoming role models.

A second Tasaru Girls Rescue Centre opened in August 2009 in Narok North district and in 2011, it hosted fifty girls, all enrolled in primary school.

Challenges

TNI's campaigns have not been smooth. Several challenges are regularly confronted, with some forming obstacles to achieving total erasure of FGM. To recap points that will by now seem familiar:

° Because the Maasai revere a culture that includes FGM, TNI has found it difficult to discuss. Most people favor it.

- Some girls who had escaped mutilation find themselves being cut during childbirth by birth attendants who are also 'circumcisers'.
- Peer pressure and the belief that fathers curse girls who refuse cutting have led many to undergo it.
- Because the community does not value female education, illiteracy is very high among the Maasai, leaving many youth unschooled and with few opportunities besides marriage.

Moreover, a girl born into a Maasai family is seen as potential wealth which might be an asset were education for women encouraged. As it is, parents marry off their daughters at an early age because the bride price, such as cows and goats, reduces poverty.

Despite FGM campaign successes, some community members remain reluctant to change. To evade the law, they perform FGM secretly and without ceremony under cover of darkness and then force daughters into hastily-arranged marriages for which they have not been prepared. For TNI, the velocity at which these events take place makes rescue an even more daunting challenge.

To overcome these obstacles, TNI hopes that:

- Continued sensitization will convince all members of the community to abandon FGM, or persuade more girls to run away and seek help.
- Engaging influential chiefs and elders in the campaign will prove to be an effective strategy.
- Making role models of Maasai girls who have run to the Centre will help convince others to refuse the practice.
- Identifying, targeting and informing 'circumcisers' and traditional birth attendants about problems caused by FGM will influence their change of heart, and
- Enforcing the law will reduce the harm.

Achievements

Despite pervasive challenges, TNI has recorded tremendous achievements that provide hope of ending FGM once and for all among the Maasai.

° TNI has engaged religious leaders in the campaign to end FGM, and pastors have taken their own initiatives to spread anti-FGM messages during Sunday services and other church functions.

° Leaders also act as community monitors, alerting the police and TNI to possible cases of FGM or early marriage. In December 2008, six girls were rescued by pastors from Free Pentecostal Church in Narok South and referred to Tasaru Girls Rescue Centre. In September 2009, another girl was saved by a pastor from her village.

° TNI trains the police on FGM, offering classes that include details of the Children's Act and international and regional instruments that protect and promote women's and children's human rights. Today in Narok, law enforcement tries to prevent the practice. Police conduct patrols within practicing communities during FGM season to warn about the risk of arrest for anyone caught carrying it out. For example, in December 2009 the station received intelligence that the neighboring Kalenjin were preparing for FGM ceremonies. Police agents, the Children's Officer and the TNI staff visited the community, reminding them that FGM is a crime and emphasizing the consequences. The community refrained, and more than 400 girls were spared.

° TNI has successfully used legislation both to prevent FGM and to prosecute. At first, TNI was reluctant to apply the lawuntil it became clear that success in community campaigns linked to the threat of punishment. 'Circumcisers' and parents have been convicted and imprisoned. As of 2011, of four FGM cases that have been referred to court, three 'circumcisers' have been prosecuted and jailed. Another father was fined 20,000 Kenyan Shillings when found guilty of organizing and marrying off his underage daughter. Similarly, when TNI rescued two girls before they were cut, the parents and 'circumciser' were arrested under section 14 of the Children's Act 2001 and charged with attempting to commit FGM. In yet another instance in which a twelve-year-old bled to death, her father and a 'circumciser' were each sentenced to ten years imprisonment. Following this judgment, elders and the local leaders led by the councilor agreed to liaise with TNI. Our association would carry out awareness interventions in Naroosora in Narok South and more specifically Enkutoto area where the tragic incident occurred. The workshops have convinced even some 'circumcisers' to denounce the practice and campaign against FGM. To ensure they do not renege on promises to stop, peer educators have monitored them. So far, no recidivism has been detected.

° The number of girls in Alternative Rites of Passage (ARP) and in school is increasing. For example, in 2009, 204 candidates underwent ARP – a rise from 137 the previous year. Now that more parents understand the consequences of FGM and have realized the importance of girls' education, they are requesting that TNI hold even more ARP trainings. Additionally, more girls at risk are running away. Between September and December 2009, Tasaru Rescue Centre received fourteen escapees from FGM and early marriage. In 2010, TNI rescued 32 girls.

° Some beneficiaries have completed secondary education and are now pursuing higher professional training courses or are working. These young women are regarded as role models in the community: successful women who have not been 'circumcised'. Their achievements have changed the perception within the community to one in which girls can also contribute to the welfare of the family.

° The Maasai had long considered FGM a taboo subject. Today, thanks to awareness workshops, numerous community members are talking about the issue and its consequences.

° Empowering young girls to say no to FGM and early marriage is slowly eroding the culture of polygamy in the Maasai community. More pupils attending and staying in school is reducing the number of under-aged second or third wives. Additionally, having graduated, teens are more aware of their rights and more likely to choose men who are not already married. The campaign also promotes respect for human rights of women and children; we are witnessing an increase in respect for their opinions and a higher value being placed on them. As increasing numbers refuse FGM and early marriage, parents have no choice but to respect their decisions.

° TNI's campaigns - along with other initiatives in the area - have made great contributions to the broader effort to end FGM in the Rift Valley provinces. According to the aforementioned KDHS survey, 2008/2009 prevalence in the region has shrunk from 42% in 2005 to 35% in 2009.

TNI will continue to work closely with villagers through peer educators who identify group entry points and establish close links. This community-friendly approach may inspire new techniques to ensure quick preventative interventions. Since men remain at present the strongest decision-makers among the Maasai, TNI has firm plans to involve men and boys in the anti-FGM campaign. After all, these boys and men, the future spouses of intact women, once involved in the process and given proper information will ensure that our efforts succeed.

TNI will also continue to provide training to the police and other law enforcement agents on issues related to FGM and early forced marriage; many girls are silently circumcised and married off but very few cases are brought to court. Law enforcement training will help achieve legal remedies.

A deep-rooted cultural practice, FGM is admittedly hard to forsake without wider community support for families. TNI's holistic approach, however, promises to hasten complete abandonment.

Notes

1 Permission to publish granted by Faiza Mohamed in Email to Tobe Levin. 5/21/2015   http://www.equalitynow.org/sites/default/files/Protecting%20Girls_ FGM_Kenya_Tanzania.pdf

2 Maasai Association website. http://www.maasai-association.org/maasai. html Retrieved 24 May 2015.

3 You will remember, however, that Kiminta is subjected to excision and infibulation.

4 Kenya Demographic and Health Survey, 2008-09, Kenya National Bureau of Statistics, Nairobi Kenya/MEASURE DHS, ICF Macro, Calverton, Maryland, USA.

5 Ibid.

With gratitude to the *International Journal of Innovation and Scientific Research* ISSN 2351-8014 Vol. 10 No. 1 Oct. 2014, pp. 40-49. © 2014 Innovative Space of Scientific Research Journals http://www.ijisr.issr-journals.org/
Corresponding Author: Peter Gutwa Oino

The essay has been edited for economy.

"The Female Genital Mutilation Act 2011 of Kenya: Challenges Facing its Implementation in Kajiado Central Sub-County, Kenya"

Geofrey Towett, Peter Gutwa Oino, and Audrey Matere

ABSTRACT: Female Genital Mutilation has been found in both developed and developing countries like Kenya. Kajiado County is one high prevalence area for girls under 13 despite FGM being a criminal offence as outlined in the Female Genital Mutilation Act of 2011. FGM continues to thrive in various parts of the country such as in Narok, Migori, Kisii, and to a larger extent Kajiado County. This paper introduces a study conducted in Kajiado Central Sub-County that examined the challenges facing effective implementation of the FGM Act of 2011. Kajiado Central Sub-County was chosen because it is largely inhabited by Maasai whose practice according to the Kenya Demographic and Health Surveys (KDHS) stands at 93 percent. This study adopted a cross sectional research design that employed various methods of data collection, i.e. using research instruments such as the semi-structured interview schedule and interview guide for Focus Group Discussions (FGDs) with traditional circumcisers, *manyatta* elders, traditional religious leaders, public health officers, and public administrative officers as well as men and women with at least five children in the study area. It found that despite the practice being criminalized with hefty penalties in Kenya, FGM is still widespread in Kajiado County where implementation of the FGM Act 2011 is constrained by a number of factors such as deeply ingrained culture and traditional behaviors, ignorance of the legislation and the consequences of FGM, anchored religious beliefs and superstition, reluctance by law enforcement officers to implement the Act as well as high poverty levels in the Sub-County. Based on the findings, this paper recommends that efforts to eliminate FGM should

° strictly enforce legislative provisions by county and national governments;
° incorporate old women and men who are the custodians of culture;
° initiate advocacy and education programs to help change the culture molders' mind sets, for instance, through the local mass media;
° initiate alternative sources of income for traditional circumcisers who depend on the practice as a source of livelihood; and
° innovate school curricula at all levels of education to incorporate themes such as female genital mutilation and its effects on the lives of girl children and women.

1 INTRODUCTION

Female Genital Mutilation is a deeply rooted historical, cultural and religious tradition that has been the subject of considerable debate.[1] Practiced for over 2,500 years in many nations but most prevalent
on the African Continent and thus considered a component of African culture, it has been classified as a critical global health issue. The custom has garnered international attention due to the political ramifications of eradication efforts and the role of the practice in

subjugating girls and women, thereby abridging their rights. The World Health Organization (WHO) defines FGM as "all procedures that involve partial or total removal of the external female genitalia, or other injury to the female genital organs for non-medical reasons."[2] In Kenya, *The Children Act* revised in 2010 defines "female circumcision" as "the cutting and removal of part or all of the female genitalia and includes the practices of clitoridectomy, excision, infibulations or other practices involving the removal of part, or of the entire clitoris or labia minora of a female person."[3] Female Genital Mutilation/Cut (FGM) is also commonly known as Female Circumcision (FC),[4] and the practice is rooted in gender inequality, in ideas about limpidness, modesty and aesthetics and in efforts to control women's sexuality. It is habitually instigated and accomplished by women who see it as a source of nobility and authority.[5] Over 140 million girls and women have experienced the cut in 27 countries in Sub-Saharan and North-East Africa, to a lesser extent in Asia and the Middle East,[6] and in Diaspora in the West. In Africa alone, United Nations organizations have estimated that up to three million girls annually are at risk.[7] In some countries FGM is inflicted as early as a few days after birth and in others as late as prior to marriage or after pregnancy. One notable trend is the progressive lowering of the age at which girls undergo the practice. A highly valued ritual, in many communities it marks the transition from childhood to womanhood[8] in rites of passage or initiation ceremonies intended to impart the skills and information it is assumed a woman will need to fulfill her duties as a wife and a mother.[9] The practice derives from varied and complex belief systems and rituals surrounding women's fertility and control of their sexuality in traditional male-dominated societies. Fran Hosken[10] contends that FGM is used by men as a tool to exercise power and govern their women. She further asserts, men claim that female sexuality is dangerous and has to be controlled.

The reasons given by communities that practice FGM vary widely but common are that it

- ° reduces sexual desire,
- ° promotes virginity and chastity,
- ° maintains fidelity among married women,
- ° promotes hygiene and
- ° creates beauty (reasoning from aesthetics).[11]

Incentives for families to continue the practice include avoiding stigma and discrimination against girls who remain intact. Considered unmarriageable and religiously 'impure', they are thought dirty and are therefore barred not only from pouring libations,[12] but also from daily activities such as cooking and community decision-making. In practicing communities such as Kisii and Kuria in Kenya, 'uncircumcised' women are viewed as 'children' - even though adult -, are banned from key social functions and denied inheritance of property. The 'bride price' (cash or kind) is also jeopardized – part of marriage transactions in African societies, generally paid to the bride's family by the groom's. Moreover, for defying ancient habits, women, like men, fear curses and ancestral wrath in communities that worship preceding generations. Furthermore, economic incentives for cutters in traditional and modern societies contribute to the practice's longevity and, in some cases, traditional practitioners' elevated status, allowing them to wield considerable power, fuel their resistance to change. Rewards for initiates, including public recognition and celebrations, gifts, the potential for marriage, respect and the ability to participate in social functions as adult women all discourage opposition. In fact, such benefits motivate some to look forward to FGM.[13]

Statistics supplied by the Kenya Demographic and Health Surveys (KDHS) show that the overall prevalence of FGM has been decreasing. In 2008/9, 27% of women in Kenya had undergone FGM, a decline from 32% in 2003 and 38% in 1998. Older women are more likely to have undergone FGM than younger ones, further indicating a decline. However, prevalence has remained highest among the Somali (97%), Kisii (96%), Kuria (96%) and the Maasai (93%);

relatively low among the Kikuyu, Kamba and Turkana, and rarely practiced among the Luo and Luhya (less than 1%).[14]

....

The Maasai ceremony – most commonly clitoridectomy – has customarily featured a large, annual celebration for all girls who have reached adolescence that year. Gathering candidates mainly between 12 and 14, groups are excised on the same day by traditional 'circumcisers' (usually experienced elderly women). Until recently, all initiates had their genitalia amputated with the same sharp instrument (often a knife called *ormurunya*) and, to stop the bleeding, a paste made from cow dung and milk fat was then applied.[15]

....

Despite the perceived socio-cultural importance that the Maasai attach to FGM, they identify complications including severe bleeding, tetanus, urinary tract infections, poor urine retention, ulceration, difficult child birth, and pain during sex.[16]

The legislative response

Female Genital Mutilation, recognized internationally as a violation of girls' and women's human rights,[17] is an act of violence that harms in many ways, limits potential for full development, and presents a major obstacle to gender equality in both developed and developing countries.

Most governments where FGM is practiced have ratified several United Nations Conventions that promote and protect females' human rights, including eliminating FGM, conventions that form part of binding international law and oblige signatory member states to protect their nationals from harmful practices such as FGM.[18]

For an up-to-date compendium of African nations with legislation against FGM, see http://www.npwj.org/FGM/Status-african-legislations-FGM.html "Status of African Legislation on FGM."

The Kenyan government has put in place several relevant policies. For instance, in 1983, the president issued a decree against FGM; on failure to stop, perpetrators were to have faced legal action. However, many communities continued in secret, inviting circumcisers to their homes without knowledge of the authorities. Thus, although the highest level of political will to eliminate FGM had been illustrated, the decree had limited success.

Following the 1993 UN Declaration on Elimination of all Forms of Violence against Women, Kenya developed a National Plan of Action for the Elimination of FGM.[19]

See National Plan of Action for the Elimination of Female Genital Mutilation in Kenya 1999–2019: https://www.k4health.org/sites/default/files/NPoA%20for%20 the%20Elimination%20of%20FGM%20inKenya.pdf. Retrieved 7 July 2015.

The UN declaration required governments to commit themselves to condemn violence against women, punish offenders, and address issues surrounding gender-based violence. This sparked even more interest in Kenya in addressing FGM, an attentiveness further reinforced by the International Conference on Population and Development (ICPD) in Cairo in 1994 and the Fourth World Conference on Women in Beijing in 1995. Following the ICPD, Kenya created a population policy known as *Sessional Paper No. 1 of 2000 on Population Policy for Sustainable Development* which advocated against FGM. Following on this achievement, the government put in place the first set of laws that dealt specifically with FGM. *The Children Act* that came into force in 2001 empowered the courts, as we have seen, to penalize those who facilitate or practice it.

While FGM declined somewhat in Kenya after implementation of *The Children Act 2001*, one in four women was still being 'cut'. This led the government to introduce a more comprehensive law, the *Prohibition of Female Genital Mutilation Act* (2011), which stipulates stiffer punishments for offenders. These include a three-to seven-year prison sentence or a fine of nearly US $6,000 for anyone practicing FGM. According to the Act, the offences punishable include aiding and abetting female genital mutilation, procuring a person to perform genital female mutilation in another country, use of premises to perform FGM, possession of tools or equipment usable in FGM, failure to report commission of offence, and use of derogatory or abusive language intended to ridicule, embarrass or otherwise harm a woman for not undergoing FGM, or a man for marrying or otherwise supporting a woman who has not undergone FGM. A person causing death by performing FGM is liable to life imprisonment.[20] The policy calls on stakeholders to take concrete steps to promote the abandonment of FGM through legislation, public education, advocacy, media coverage, the empowerment of women, and access to reproductive health and other support services. These laws and policies are supported by the 2010 Constitution of Kenya, which reaffirms the government's commitment to protect and promote human rights and fundamental freedoms.[21]

It should be noted nonetheless that despite the enactment and implementation of the FGM Act of 2011 as well as a new constitution in 2010, prevalence remains high, especially for the Maasai, standing at 93% (among females of 13-49 years). It is against this background, therefore, that the researchers sought to uncover challenges facing effective implementation of the FGM Act of 2011 in Kenya's Kajiado Central Sub-County.

2 RESEARCH METHODOLOGY

The study was conducted in 2012 in Kajiado Central Sub-County, population 687,312, in an area of 21,292.7 km square. Kajiado County as a whole is largely occupied by the Maasai community. Kajiado Central Sub-County consists of fourteen wards with a population of 48,800 inhabitants. It is one of the three sub-counties of Kajiado County that share common borders with Nairobi County, Machakos

County and Kiambu County.[22] We chose to focus on Kajiado Central Sub-County because it is dominated by the Maasai community known both locally and internationally for its conservative lifestyle, traditions and culture, and the Sub-County has experienced violent protests by pro-FGM campaigners against government officers and the local populace who oppose the 'cut'. The pro-FGM advocates have been women drawn from various wards in the Sub-County.

We adopted a cross sectional research design. Four out of fourteen wards were randomly sampled and a sample size of 200 respondents was used to solicit data. Respondents comprised traditional circumcisers, *manyatta* elders, traditional religious leaders, public health officers, administrative officers from the sampled wards and sampled men and women with at least five children in the study area. Data was collected via semi-structured interviews and Focus Group Discussions.

The paper focuses primarily on the challenges facing effective implementation of the FGM Act of 2011 of Kenya.

3 FINDINGS AND DISCUSSION

The subsequent sections highlight the discussion of major findings.

3.1 CHALLENGES CONSTRAINING EFFECTIVE IMPLEMENTATION OF FGM ACT 2011

The researchers sought to uncover the challenges facing effective implementation of the FGM Act of 2011 in Kajiado Central Sub-County. ... 110 respondents (55%) attributed non-compliance to deeply embedded culture, while 12 (6%) attributed it to reluctance by law enforcement officers who are implementers of the policy. In addition, 48 (24%) cited entrenched religious beliefs and superstition while 8 (4%) attributed it to the high poverty level in the region. Finally, the findings also indicated that 22 respondents (11%) cited ignorance of the legislation and the consequences of FGM as a constraining factor to implementation.

3.1.1 DEEPLY INGRAINED MAASAI CULTURE AND TRADITION

Our findings showed that the leading factor constraining effective implementation of the policy is deep-rooted Maasai culture and tradition. 55% of respondents held that ... marriage and ancestral relationship consider FGM essential in the rite of passage demanded of girls over age 13 who must be 'officially' initiated into society. One female respondent illustrated a typical attitude by insisting that "uncircumcised girls are indecent because they are promiscuous, ever sex-hungry and never have stable families. They are like cars without brakes and are absolutely, sexually uncontrollable. HIV/AIDS is never far from their doorstep. Furthermore, they can neither fetch wealth to the parents nor get a marriage partner in the community. They are just cursed ..." (Female, age 46).

The Maasai community despises females accused of promiscuity but believes that FGM obviates the reviled behavior. In addition, giving daughters in marriage once they are 'circumcised' guarantees family wealth. Hence, the cultural value of FGM can also be measured in number of cows, sheep and goats the parents receive as bride price, another strong incentive to uphold excision at all cost.

The findings further unearthed the Maasai conviction that uncircumcised women are ever 'young girls' who can never 'grow up'. As one female respondent explained, "The Maasai celebrate FGM because community secrets regarding the institution of marriage are passed on. ... [Girls learn] good behavior and responsibility in marriage and thus ... failure of responsibility among women is reduced. Which *moran* in our community would like to marry an uncircumcised girl who knows nothing regarding such community secrets?" (Female, age 42 years). Marriage, family and economics give FGM a significant role, hence endearing the practice to community opinion-leaders. ...

Furthermore, resistance to the FGM Act 2011 drew strongly on Maasai identity. In contrast to other communities, the group sees itself affirming 'ways' that include 'circumcision'. An individual sees him or herself as a Maasai largely based on this rite which confirms a sense of belonging. They therefore maintain that FGM must be continued and eradication efforts resisted at all cost. ...

Identity, however, isn't the only determinant in failure to enforce the law. Practical measures kick in, too. One administrative officer argued that the Maasai's nomadic lifestyle impedes enforcement. The tribe migrates constantly, often to Tanzania. As the officer quipped, "It's hard apprehending perpetrators in search of pasture and water. ... Before our officers are mobilized, they are already past the border and don't come back to the same spot when they return. They settle elsewhere and continue the practice and thus, trans-border migration provides safe hiding from the law" (Male, age 37). ...

3.1.2 IGNORANCE OF LEGISLATION AND CONSEQUENCES OF FGM

Research findings indicated that 11 percent of respondents attributed failure in compliance to ignorance of the legislation as well as the consequences of FGM. Seventy-two percent, – largely *manyatta* elders, traditional religious leaders and men and women sampled for the study –, were illiterate and unaware of possible criminal proceedings. Although public health officers and administrators in charge of various locations and sub-locations in the sampled wards were fully informed, they admitted that illiteracy and lack of awareness-raising campaigns had largely contributed to the continued existence of FGM in the community. When researchers urged a female respondent to say more about her knowledge of the law and its provisions, she replied, "I can't read or write, let alone understand the content of that document. Women in our community learn through informal means such as teachings after the 'cut'. It is surely news to hear that … our most valued rite has been prohibited. Nobody ever asked us our opinion before coming up with such a repressive law and I, therefore, find it unacceptable to us" (Female, age 44). …

According to J. Anderson (in *Public Policymaking*, 2nd edition. NY: Holt, Rinehart & Winston, 1978), legislation that is largely inconsistent with culture and traditions often faces considerable non-compliance in both developed and developing countries. A female public health officer – Maasai –, on further questioning by our researchers, admitted, "The community I come from still holds that FGM is important since it reduces complications during childbirth, lowers promiscuity, contributes to cleanliness in the genital area and avoids disease. … Efforts to teach negative consequences have never yielded fruit since most of the elites including myself and many learned women underwent the cut" (Female, age 31).

This response suggests that most community members remain ignorant of the negative consequences of FGM, believing instead that cutting is paramount in keeping women clean, permitting easy child birth and limiting disease. Known health risks posed by FGM contradict this – such as death due to excessive bleeding, hemorrhage, post-operative shock, fractures of the clavicle or dislocation of the hip joint if heavy pressure is applied to restrain the struggling girl, infection as a result of unhygienic conditions, clitoral neuroma, calculus formation in the vagina and more. …

3.1.3 INGRAINED TRADITIONAL RELIGIOUS BELIEFS AND SUPERSTITION

As indicated above, a total of 48 respondents (24%) attributed non-compliance to ingrained religious beliefs and superstition. The Maasai are monotheistic, worshipping a single deity called *Enkai* who sends each person a guardian spirit to watch over her or him from birth to death. The guardian spirit, it is believed, brings great blessings to all who abide by Maasai culture and tradition but delivers calamities and death to renegades and turncoats who reveal the community's best guarded secrets – of which "circumcision" is one. During an interview, a traditional religious leader (*Loonki-dongi*) stated, "Blessed be Enkai who brings good fortune to the faithful and destroys his enemies. Enkai values true Maasai who abide by our customs and tradition. He, however, curses the rebels and traitors by bringing death to the community. He can send the red cock (lightning), to strike individuals who rebel, or death among the *morans* during cattle raids" (Male, aged 52).

Researchers' further querying revealed that, according to this religious leader, death is attributed to rebellion against culture and tradition and, thus, appeasement must be made to calm both the ancestors and the irritated guardian. Such mollification is achieved when libation is poured and a sacrificial lamb is offered. He argued moreover that during both male and female 'circumcision', the blood that is shed, a sign of absolute spiritual devotion, calms the ancestral spirits and guardian angel. The initiated boys and girls consequently take an oath never to reveal community secrets including talking about circumcision in public or to the uncircumcised within and outside the Maasai group. As one manyatta elder quipped, "Female circumcision is our culture. Why should we be forced to abandon it when we were born into it? Abandoning our culture would annoy our ancestors and bring a community curse" (Male, age 55).

The study found that the Maasai attribute various occurrences such as disability, neonatal death, skin diseases, lightning strikes, death during cattle raids and barrenness to abandonment of Maasai culture and traditions. For instance, a newborn may die if a woman is not 'circumcised' since the guardian spirit is angry at the mother. Excised women are believed to give birth more easily because 'circumcision' not only appeased the ancestors and the guardian spirit by shedding blood but also prepared the birth canal for the infant's passage. Thus, enemies of FGM, we found, are harbingers of calamity to be fought in public and cursed by elders who call on intruders to die mysterious deaths. Such unquestioned religious beliefs and superstition in the Sub-County have indeed largely constrained implementation of the 2011 FGM Act.

3.1.4 RELUCTANCE BY LAW ENFORCEMENT OFFICERS

According to Section 2(d) of the FGM Act 2011, law enforcement – comprising police, the provincial administration, children's officers, probation, gender, social development and cultural officers – has a role to play in addressing FGM. This research established that six percent (6%) of respondents believed the police, especially local officers, have largely been reluctant to enforce the law. One respondent, himself a location chief, said, "Law enforcement officers, especially the chiefs and sub-chiefs, have witnessed unprecedented hostility from community members after trying to implement the Act. A sub-chief from my precinct had his house razed to the ground by an angry group of women. Other law enforcement agents including health officers have since been threatened should they ever try to rebel against the culture and tradition of their community" (Male, 59).

Sub-chiefs and chiefs in their respective areas of jurisdiction have in fact faced enormous aggression in efforts to stop the rite. Though there appears to be goodwill toward implementing the Act on the part of law enforcement, extreme opposition – for instance, arson -- had prompted them to go slow with implementation in their jurisdictions. In addition, other officials such as health officers who tried to communicate the consequences of the 'cut' had been considered traitors and rebels against the community's most treasured cultural practice. Such antagonism has influenced public officers' reluctance to apply the Act.

In this regard, we augmented this study with evidence from various sources including media outlets that also report aggressive opposition to abolition. For instance, on June 3, 2014, the *Kenyan Standard* reported serious injuries inflicted by infuriated women in Kajiado County accusing reporters of opposing FGM. The newspaper noted that

... Three journalists including a writer were injured and ... treated at a nearby health centre after the demonstrators turned to them accusing them for being at the forefront in fighting FGM. NTV Cameraman Mr Abdalah Ngotho and Ms Christine Musa of Media Max were injured during the melee while Mr Ngotho's television camera was damaged. As whipping went on, Media-Max's Christine opted to save herself using the Maasai dialect declaring she is circumcised and advocating for FGM, too. Unfortunately the irate women demanded to strip her off for inspection to ascertain her truth (*Standard* [newspaper], 4 June 2014. p. 2).

The report captured one instance of aggression against journalists in the county, but, in fact, fighting against public officials often occurs and goes unreported as such because, if publicized, the news would embarrass the victims and elicit their fear that the bad publicity would bring further reprisals on chiefs, sub-chiefs or various public health officers. Silence has therefore been preferred together with reluctance to follow up on reported cases of FGM – one more element impeding efforts to eradicate FGM in the Sub-County.

3.1.5 HIGH POVERTY LEVEL

Our findings revealed that resistance to implementing the FGM Act 2011 was also attributed to various stakeholders' economic gain, as suggested by four percent (4%) of respondents. Focus group discussion disclosed that key actors who mostly benefit economically from FGM include traditional circumcisers, religious leaders, initiates' parents and a few law enforcement officers bribed to keep silent. Moreover, parents greatly value the practice since it fetches a lot of cows and goats when the girl is finally given over to marriage. Young men who wed a 'circumcised' woman are required to pay up to seventy cows plus twenty sheep and goats as bride price, thereby bringing considerable wealth to the bride's parents. Rather than investing in girls' education, Maasai stress FGM. In a focus group, one village elder pointed out how "most members of the community [base] their economic status on the number of livestock they get as bride price, not on the western education that degrades African culture. Having more girls in a family means wealth in waiting since they fetch a lot of cows and goats when they are circumcised and given over to marriage" (Female, age 48).

The study further established that, in places where the practice is popular and entrenched, traditional circumcisers are highly revered.

Paid based on the number of initiates they cut, excisers have a specific interest in promoting what they do and hence often claim that ancestors and guardian spirits watching over the community will punish the homes of those who challenge a practice passed down from the great grandparents. Since fear of curse among the Maasai assures continued high reverence for traditional circumcisers, the community often follows their instructions as absolute truth and they, in turn, do everything to promote this aspect of their culture and resist its eradication. Owing to the high poverty level in Kajiado County, most community members but especially religious leaders, circumcisers, some public officers and parents defend 'circumcision' as both an avenue to economic gain and a cultural rite worth protecting. Such community gate-keepers maintain that efforts to eradicate FGM should be resisted at all cost knowing that, for some, cutting constitutes a major strand of income.

4 CONCLUSION AND RECOMMENDATIONS

The foregoing discussion reveals that FGM is considered by some to be an outdated custom that has rightly been criminalized in Kenya. However, it is still widely practiced in Kajiado Central Sub-County in Kajiado County. Kenya effected the FGM Act of 2011 to eradicate the practice; however, efforts have achieved little impact and have been largely hampered by ingrained Maasai culture and tradition, ignorance of the legislation and consequences of FGM, strong traditional religious beliefs and superstition, reluctance by law enforcement to implement the Act as well as high poverty levels in the Sub-County, which have influenced the initiators to continue the practice as a way of generating income for themselves and their families. Based on the findings of the study, this paper recommends that efforts to eliminate FGM should not only be backed up by strictly enforcing legislative provisions by the county and national governments, but also by incorporating both old women and men who are custodians of culture in the Maasai community. At the same time, the stakeholders should initiate advocacy and education programs to help change the culture holders' mind-sets, for instance, through local mass media.

Additionally, there is need to assure alternative sources of income for traditional circumcisers who depend on the practice for their livelihood. Finally, school curricula, at all educational levels, should incorporate themes such as female genital mutilation and its effects on the lives of girl children and women.

References

1   See Farnoosh Rezaee Ahan. (2012) "Theories on Female Genital Mutila-tion." Uppsala: Department of Cultural Anthropology, Uppsala University. http://www.researchgate.net/profile/Farnoosh_Milde_Rezaeeahan/publication/256058457_Theories_on_Female_Genital_Mutilation/links/00b4952add1b8b38c9000000.pdf. Retrieved 8 July 2015.

2   World Health Organization (2008). *Eliminating Female Genital Mu-tilation: An interagency statement.* OHCHR, UNAIDS, UNDP, UN-ECA, UNESCO, UNFPA, UNHCR, UNICEF, UNIFEM, WHO. Geneva. http://www.un.org/womenwatch/daw/csw/csw52/statements_missions/Inter-agency_Statement_on_Eliminating_FGM.pdf Retrieved 8 July 2015.

3   Laws of Kenya. *The Children Act.* Chapter 141. Revised Edition 2010 (2007). Published by the National Council for Law Reporting with the Authority of the Attorney General. www.kenyalaw.org
https://www.icrc.org/applic/ihl/ihl-nat.nsf/a24d1cf3344e99934125673e00508142/95bcf642e7784b63c1257b4a004f95e8/$FILE/Children%27s%20Act.pdf. Retrieved 8 July 2015.

4   United Nations Children's Fund. (2008) *Coordinated Strategy to Abandon Female Genital Mutilation/cutting in One Generation: A human rights-based approach to programming,* Technical Note, UNICEF. NY.

5   Nussbaum, M. (1999) *Sex and Social Justice.* Oxford: Oxford UP.

6   UNICEF (2013). *Female Genital Mutilation/cutting: A statistical overview and exploration of the dynamics of change.* New York. http://www.unicef.org/publi-cations/index_69875.html. Retrieved 8 July 2015.

7   United Nations. 2012. *Advancement of Women: Report of the Third Committee.* http://daccess-dds-ny.un.org/doc/UNDOC/GEN/N13/603/90/PDF/N1360390.pdf?OpenElement. Retrieved 8 July 2015.

8   Appropriate Technology in Health (PATH) (1999). *Female Genital Circumci-sion in Four Districts in Kenya.* Nairobi.

9   United States Department of State. *Kenya: Report on Female Genital mutila-tion (FGM) or Female Genital Cutting (FGC),* 1 June 2001. Available at: http://www.refworld.org/docid/46d5787932.html Retrieved 8 July 2015.

10 Hosken, Fran P. (1993). *The Hosken Report: Genital and Sexual Mutilation of Females.* 4th Revised Edition. Women's International Network News: Lexington, MA.

11 Dorkenoo, E. (1994) *Cutting the Rose – Female Genital Mutilation: The prac-tice and its prevention.* London: Minority Rights Group.

12 Hicks, E. K. (1993). *Infibulation: Female Mutilation in Islamic Northeastern Africa.* New Brunswick, NJ: Transaction Books.

13 Hosken, *Ibid.*

14 Government of Kenya (GOK). (1998). *Kenya Demographic and Health Survey* (KDHS). Nairobi: Government of Kenya.

15 Arhem, K. *The Maasai and the State: The Impact of Rural Development Policies on a Pastoral People in Tanzania,* Discussion Paper No. 52 at IWGIA.

http://www.iwgia.org/publications/search-pubs?publication_id=170 Retrieved 8 July 2015.

16 Berntsen, John L. (1977) *Maasai and lloikop: Ritual Experts and Their Followers*. African Studies Program. University of Wisconsin.

17 Rahman, A. and Toubia, N. (2000) *Female Genital Mutilation: A Guide to Laws and Policies Worldwide*. London: Zed.

18 Ibid.

19 Mohamed, Faiza. (2011) *Protecting girls from undergoing Female Genital Mutilation: The Experience of Working with the Maasai Communities in Kenya and Tanzania*. See http://www.equalitynow.org/sites/default/files/Protecting%20Girls_FGM_Kenya_Tanzania.pdf. Retrieved 7 July 2015.

20 The Prohibition of Female Genital Mutilation Act, 2011 No. 32 of 2011. https://www.k4health.org/sites/default/files/NPoA%20for%20the%20Elimination%20of%20FGM%20inKenya.pdf. Retrieved 7 July 2015.

21 Government of Kenya (2010) *The Constitution of Kenya*. Nairobi: Government Printers.

22 Gwako, L. (1992) *Female Circumcision in Kenya: A Study of Gusii Women Experience and Current Attitude With Implication for Social Change.*

Eldoret, Kenya: Moi University.

Reflections on Kiminta's Tale

Valentine Nkoyo

Kiminta's story has given me a friend, a sister, a true African warrior with whom I not only share the experience of FGM but also the passion to defend the vulnerable and speak out openly, affirming pride in our good traditions yet agreeing to abandon the harmful. Customs that inflict suffering and violate human rights should end. Kiminta prays, "May the Maasai conserve their rich culture, retain ceremonial rituals, continue feasting and blessing initiates, but cease amputating women's sex." I couldn't agree more!

I love my culture very much as it gave me an identity! In fact, I can't imagine any people bereft of admirable qualities. Deprived of our beneficent traditions, I would feel like an empty shell!

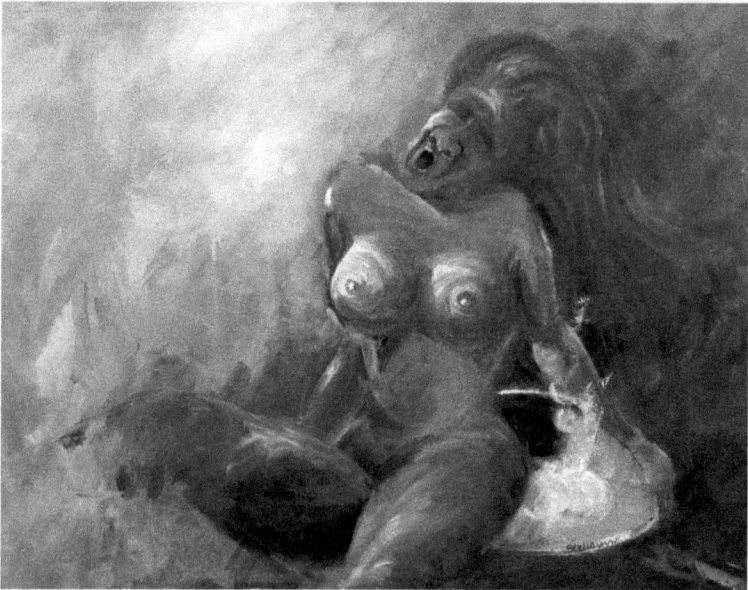

Stella Ubigho. "Agony – An Experience I Will Never Forget" (Oil on Canvas, 1998)

Therefore, although born female where educating girls is frowned upon, I know who I am and value our uniqueness as Maasai, apart from those few practices that cause trauma and contravene rights.

You may sense a discrepancy here – pride and abjection – but Kiminta, too, implies that ethnic honor feeds the courage "to liberate children" from the culture's "emotional bondage." My passion to make a difference, like Kiminta's, is based on the horrifying experience of FGM which is not, as some may argue, an integral part of being Maasai. I can be Maasai even if intact!

And once assured of this, I can mute the throwback to my own 'event' that Kiminta vividly evokes. Her description of that day squeezes the heart. So well written, it makes her kin to other girls whose detailed memories echo hers. Absolutely typical, the chronicle underscores the inexorability of pain, its details stubborn and greedy.

Most survivors vividly remember what they endured, the *mutilation* of their genitals. Unless they cut you as an infant, you *cannot* forget the brutal ripping off of flesh -- while robust arms pin you down, ensuring you don't fight back, and your captors belt out earsplitting songs, guaranteeing that no one hears you scream. Meaning, don't think there's anyone to rescue you!

How could you not recall, especially when the night before you were scared to death and had no idea to whom to run?
Or if you dared to flee, the question was, where to?
And if you ran away, could you ever come back?
How would you face the shame you had put your parents to?

And by the way, your evasion would be carved in stone, the story of your flight told again and again to other young rebellious girls, not to encourage mimicry but to terrify them at all costs.

How could you disremember if you were petrified of stigma and anticipated disrespect and mockery, labeled the 'dirty' girl, the coward, the 'spinster', the traitor?

Who wants to be cast out from among her own?

And how do you suppress the memory of an assault that causes not only instant anguish but also continues infecting your entire life?

Kiminta's words – "When I was growing up in Kenya, I had a single option, to become someone's wife" – summarizes how much weight our culture puts on marriage. Marriageability is so significant that any hindrance concerns not only the family but also the community at large.

Yes, perceptions are changing but slowly. When I was cut about 20 years ago, men wouldn't dare take an "uncut" bride. Had they done so, their egos would have suffered; the laughing stock among their peers, they would have been judged "awkward." Today, however, some grooms reject "cut" girls and tell their parents so – but not yet in numbers large enough to make a difference. The critical mass has yet to be reached. Deeply rooted in their culture, people with entrenched interests in the multiple aspects of the custom remain unwilling to relinquish it. One reason surely lies outside the act itself. For many years the Maasai have resisted change while observing alteration in communities surrounding them.

Their resistance can be fierce. In 2014 in Kenya, over 3,000 Maasai women gathered in the bushes to oppose the government's mandate to end FGM.[1] A few months later, campaigners and police were attacked for intervening.[2] In fact, a few educated speakers, exuding confidence, denounced the kind of 'outsider' meddling that claimed 'universal human rights' were on its side. Such appeals wouldn't stop *them* from performing FGM.

If schooling and awareness-raising fail, then I advocate deploying the full force of the law, for in a nation like Kenya where FGM has been declared illegal, legislation should be applied. Government must be held accountable when regimes shirk their duty to protect the vulnerable young, the future leaders of coming generations!

Yes, inflammable topics demand sensitivity, and every effort should be taken to avoid backlash. This is best accomplished by empowering survivors, community leaders and youth, encouraging them to get involved.

My experience of FGM

Thinking about it now, I find unfathomable, truly unbelievable, the tidal wave of helplessness that overwhelmed me when told in Maasai by my mother, "Iyiolo ajo etaa iaku enkitok?" meaning "Do you know it's time you became a woman?"

I was only eleven years old when she broke the news.

The whole village gathered and, amid dancing and singing, we girls were taken to a clearing in the bush. With the neighbors on my right, I had my sister to the left. Chosen to go first, she was to set an example for me.

The very instant I reclined, they sprang, pinning down my arms and legs. My eyes snapped shut. But darkness failed to block the noise of my sister's struggles. "Keep still!" the women ordered.

She did. The thrashing stopped, and not a single sound escaped her lips. I then opened my eyes only to find terror in the form of the old lady moving swiftly on to me. My lids plummetted again but not fast enough to blot out that face I still see before me now, those long earlobes with ornaments and a hand with the razor. Each and every movement of that blade searing through my flesh slicing me to pieces – I felt and remember it all.

Every time the assault enters my thoughts, so do her nose, her cheeks, her grimness, those facial features of the thief who stole what had been mine, what had been ME, filching something vital to my life.

"Nnyo amu itaa enkitok."

"Get up! You are a woman now," she ordered after the ordeal. A nightmare! Something meant to be "good" for me had been so appalling that describing it most of the time ends in tears. ...

The following weeks saw the frequent use of Dettol, a disinfectant I hate even now as it reminds me of how helpless the blade made me feel. True, the herbs used to prevent infection and hasten healing worked to some extent, yet intense pain remained. I feared to urinate let alone stand the sting of salty water, disinfectants and the herbs.

For weeks afterward, I remember hating even to approach the place where we were cut. One day, though, I gathered my strength and returned, hoping to recuperate something I had lost even though I didn't know what it was. The blood stains were still there but no flesh. Had what they chopped off us fed birds or beasts? The thought upset me.

For more than a decade and a half, I couldn't stand to talk about FGM. If people raised the issue, I would simply leave. For quite some time I was distressed but not angry at anyone in particular. My understanding for many years had been that what I was made to go through served to "fit" me into the community and would allow me to get a husband. Otherwise, no one would marry me. As a teen, however, I had started questioning the reasons behind FGM and doubting the excuses people gave for it.

My change of heart came in 2013. Then I started being vocal about FGM, especially after all the media attention. Because the Maasai became known for fighting to keep it going, friends kept asking me if I had endured it. A difficult period followed; ambivalent and confused, I didn't want to come out and so would say nothing or even deny that it had been done to me.

I started feeling very bad, however, for ignoring the issue and living in denial.

In 2014, I registered the Mojatu Foundation to allow me to work closely with women and young people, mainly girls. I aim to inspire other survivors to share their stories and, by getting involved, to break the silence around FGM. Openness alone can improve the chances of girls at risk.

As a female born into patriarchal culture, I also suffered an on-going fight for education. In desperation when confronted with an impending child marriage –my own–, and unable to convince my father using logic, I drafted a poem in my mother tongue to appeal to his emotions, pleading with him to educate me. I touched his better nature; in fact, he wept and complied.

The joy of bringing education to others and empowering those most vulnerable --especially girls and women -- is my passion. Eradicating FGM in a generation is a life commitment I made, and I am working towards that aim in partnership with others.

Like Kiminta, I had to move on in life. To safeguard those at risk and offer comfort to survivors, my choice, too, was speaking out.

Experience turned into positive action

Since registering Mojatu Foundation, we have …
- ° Mobilised and started the FGM Steering group with over 30 members from over 23 countries and I chair the group;

- ° Tasked a member (community representative) of the Nottinghamshire City and County FGM Strategy Board to develop an FGM referral pathway;
- ° Run community magazines working mainly with African and Caribbean communities. (See www.issuu.com/mojatu and www.issuu.com/mojatuberks for the last few years.)
- ° Organized a national conference in February 2015 that brought more than 85 people together;
- ° Trained and managed 12 Community Media Champions reporting on issues affecting communities – mainly girls and omen -- with a focus on FGM;
- ° Presented at numerous local, national and international conferences or workshops – including at Lady Margaret Hall, University of Oxford on March 7, 2015 – and local and national media houses, mainly on FGM and issues affecting marginalized women;
- ° Been signposting and referring survivors and children at risk to relevant services;
- ° Supported over 34 volunteers with 5 girls currently training in graphic design, web development and maintenance;
- ° Worked and continue working with other organizations to develop a sports and leadership scheme for girls and women;
- ° Launched an FGM survivors' club in Nottingham.

In sum, raising professionals' awareness of FGM in healthcare, social work and education is not easy, but altering perceptions among hardcore adherents presents an even greater challenge. Still, a rights-based approach to change people's minds will win the battle in the end.

FGM should be everybody's business!

I dream of the day when the razors drop. It can't come soon enough!

For further details visit <www.valentinenkoyo.com> and <www. mojatu.com>.

Endnotes

1 K24TV (2014). "Over 3,000 Maasai Women Meet In Kajiado To Campaign For The 'Cut'." <https://www.youtube.com/watch?v=VAqthu7uN2c>. Retrieved 4 May 2015.

2 NTV (2014). "We Want the Cut! Kilgoris women demonstrate, attack anti-FGM activists." <https://www.youtube.com/watch?v=Zw_H6K3pJBs>. Retrieved 3 May 2015.

Critique of Anthr/apologists observing a Maasai rite

Tobe Levin

[FGM] is an affront to human dignity, an assault on health and an impediment to the well-being of families, communities and countries. Human development cannot be fully achieved as long as women and girls ... suffer from this human rights violation or live in fear of it.

Dr. Babatunde Osotimehin, Director of UNFPA qtd. in Siddharth Chatterjee

On November 26, 2014, a court in Kilgoris, Kenya, condemned 19-year-old Faith Tanui to three years in prison or a fine of 200,000 Kenyan shillings – a sum punitively high. Her crime? Having recently undergone excision apparently at her own request, she was on trial for "having failed to report the commission of FGM."[1] The misdeed took place in Kilibwet village and the trial in Trans Mara East Sub County – a region largely populated by Maasai.

Among comments following the online feature, one critical respondent, Oloo Macharia reminds us how imbricated in colonial resentment the excision issue can be. Suggesting that the Kenyan government acted "for the pleasure of foreigners" (... "are we afraid that they may not bribe us with loans and grants which they eventually take back with usury, anyway?") s/he demands:

Let those who cut do it. Let those who don't cut - not cut. Should it cease serving our cultural/religious purposes, FGM and/or MGM practices will die a natural death, with time and without regime intervention. It is inadvisable to tamper with practices which have evolved over centuries and generations. ... Our ancestors ... were not evil. ... For some of us, both our parents were cut. Is there anything wrong with us? Government out of our genitals![2]

This broadly propagated viewpoint credits outside pressure with African regimes' embrace of bodily integrity.

Yet FGM is, and has always been, an African issue long before anyone opposed it in the West. Consider the examples of Babibkar Badri, Marie Asaad, Dr. Nawal el Saadawi, Dr. Irene Thomas, Dr. Olayinka Koso-Thomas, Dr. Asma el Dareer, Edna Adan, the late Efua Dorkenoo OBE, Dr. Morissanda Kouyate, Berhane Ras-Work, Awa Thiam, Khady Koita, Comfort Momoh, Comfort Ottah, the Inter-African Committee represented in 28 African nations plus scores of additional veteran activists who insisted – at a symposium at the University of Dakar in 1982, for instance – that my own reporting should correct this erroneous belief.

Opposition to FGM had never been an exclusive colonial import. On the contrary, as Awa Thiam insists in *Warrior Marks*, human rights emerge from indigenous African values.

The fact of female dissidence in cutting cultures notwithstanding, equally injudicious now is any effort, in an increasingly globalized world, to disentangle 'pristine' 'African' points of view from perspectives on Africa expressed by the Diaspora. For instance, on June 20, 2015, in Geneva, Dr. Pierrette Herzberger-Fofana, President of FORWARD –Germany, received the African Woman in Europe 2015 prize for humanitarian engagement. AWE (African Women in Europe) offered the award, suggesting that fighting FGM – the explicit mandate of FORWARD - Germany – belongs in the repertoire of honorable actions elevating African women's prestige.[3]

Thus, when Kiminta proposed a book based on her experience, I was keen to add her voice to the increasing number of Africans, women and men, who execrate the cut. A Maasai resident in Germany, Kiminta bravely describes her challenge by blade and thus, authorized as a cultural insider, blows the whistle on FGM.[4]

As her amanuensis, I draw inspiration from my first encounter with the custom, a journalist's rendering offered by *EMMA*, the German feminist magazine. In its third issue, April 1977 – yes, that long ago – Pauline Caravello headlined her article "Clitoridectomy," the bold type booming from the double page spread. "What's that?" I asked, along with the magazine's 150,000 other readers. Once we knew, FGM never let us go. A movement sprang up in Germany, with numbers that have waxed and waned, but in the early 90s,

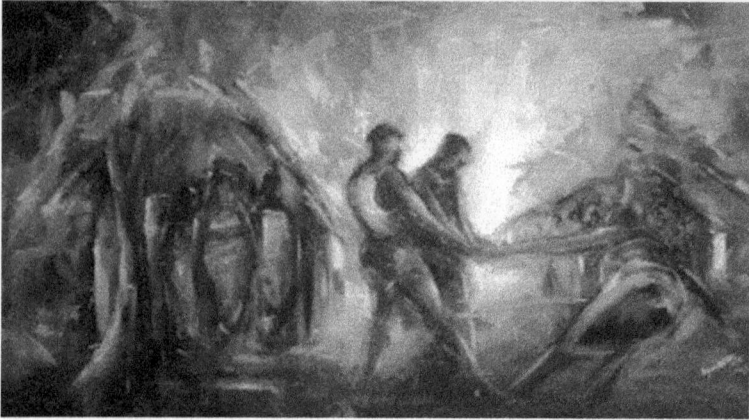

Manasseh Imonikebe. "What If I Refuse?" (Oil on Canvas, 1998)

it expanded, and at present Germany hosts more than 30 groups against FGM, nearly all of them networking together under the umbrella forum INTEGRA. This fascinating history cannot, of course, be told here, but the journalist's concluding plea moves us to this day. Based on interviews with informants in Khartoum, Caravello cites a Sudanese woman who implored, "Here nobody talks about infibulation. Families are silent; the media, too. We [campaigners who want to see the torture end] are appealing for an outcry from abroad. Tell the world …"[5]

What then is the world to know?

Commanded to lie down, the child is forcibly restrained; her hands are immobilized and legs are trussed. The sufferer highlights these arrangements, suggesting anticipation of resistance. In Imonikebe Manasseh's oil, "What If I Refuse?" (1998) we see what the instigators' subterfuge and brutal measures wanted to avoid.[6]

Next, with fetters now in place, groping in haste at the crux of the little girl's being, the exciser nails the clitoris and slashes it, presenting the fresh flesh to "senior female relatives" for approval of the quantity removed. Enough? her gesture asks.

When ululations affirm the booty, the aggressor wields the blade again, now capturing the lips while Kiminta howls and bleeds.

Then she is stitched and the wound dressed with raw egg and herbs until "the brew," as she tells us "augmented by [her] blood, [can] crust..."

This is what it is and yet ... only now, four decades after a global movement began, is the truth coming out. As Virginia Woolf wrote in *A Room of One's Own*, women's advancement can be chronicled only together with men's resistance to it. Applied to campaigns to stop FGM, they can be written only together with efforts to suppress them.

One of many insidious attempts recently came to my attention. On July 18, 2014, *The Nairobian* headline announced: "Traditionalist: Female Genital Operation is holy, biblically and culturally."

John Arap Koech, chair of Sorun Amabet (save before it gets lost) dedicated to preserving Kalenjin culture including "female circumcision," "has sworn to defend the outlawed Female Genital Mutilation through thick and thin, because it is 'holy' biblically and culturally."[7] When in Kajiado Maasai women demonstrated against criminalizing FGM, Koech travelled there to defend them.

Challenging the validity of the General Assembly's resolution to "Ban FGM Worldwide" (20 December 2012), he has written the United Nations petitioning to revoke it. Claiming exaggeration of the custom's harms, he accuses the convocation of bias because the drafters failed to "engage or consult 'stakeholders' before outlawing the practice." It was, however, the African caucus itself that had proposed the measure. Nonetheless, "the traditionalist blames British missionaries whom he accuses of colonizing many parts of Africa in 1885 and weakening local communities' cultures through formal education and Christianity."[8]

The call to dispense with formal education notwithstanding, it is true that the Church has a record of mixed results in historical efforts to stop FGM. In the sixteenth century, for instance, Jesuits in Ethiopia (then Abyssinia) demanded that converts cease cutting.

Yet
> ... the men refused to marry women who were not excised and [therefore] conversions stopped. At the urgent advice of the Pope, the Church, "preferring souls to sexual organs" (as Benoîte Groult so graphically put it in her book *Ainsi Soit-Elle)*, sanctioned the practice as "medically necessary." Fran Hosken, a U.S. feminist who helped initiate international concern over female mutilation, reports that since then all Catholic missions have permitted the procedure on daughters of converts.[9]

The acceptance of FGM that emerges above – indigenous majorities defend it, as do practitioners even in the modern sector with their own vested interests – allies with another, less defensible defense, this time by scholars who, I can't help but add, ought to know better. In fact, they DO know better ...

Let's consider a fairly typical example, the report of an anthr/ apologist who has studied the Maasai. I've taken Aud Talle's field notes, rearranged and condensed them to improve readability but kept in quotation marks the exact words she chose.

Whereas Kiminta endures the abuse, Talle watches an older Maasai girl rebel.

"As soon as the circumciser began cutting her flesh," Talle reports, "the [teen] started to fight back." When attendants failed "to hold her down … the elder brother and guardian … told [them] … to use ropes."[10]

The operation had to take place at once "because the cattle were restlessly waiting." But things were taking time. Efforts to lasso the girl's ankles failed because, desperate, she kicked and struggled until exhaustion claimed her and she could finally be bound.

Yet it's not straight sailing yet. Without room in which to wrench her thighs apart, the actors called for back-up, and it came.

> One of the men observing the scene … offer[ed to] help. Forcing his stick through the mud wall …, he made a hole, and pulled out one of the rope ends. The other rope was fastened to a roof beam at the entrance to the house (94-95).[11]

The two paragraphs with this crucial information about ropes and bondage cover one entire page in Talle's chapter, for attention is diverted from the action by interventions clarifying, from the perpetrators' point of view, each step. The effect is to dilute the impact of what is actually happening: violence criminalized by most nation's laws and international covenants. But to get back to the point:

> At last, the circumciser could proceed. … With tiny movements she carved away the clitoris and the labia minora, while the women in loud voices instructed her how to cut. The blood rushed forward, and for us outside the actual scene, it was as if the excited voices of the women and the heavy breathing of the girl would never … end. (95)

But wait! I tell myself. If the observer is outside, how does she know about these 'tiny movements'? How can she discern what's cut? In fact, she "peeped through [an] opening in the roof that the women had made beforehand to lighten up the room" (95). And spying with her are kids of both sexes, not to mention the volunteer male who is "all the time holding tightly to the rope [while gazing] into the narrow room to check that the women did a proper job" (95). Excuse me? The man observes to assess the cutter's skill?

In any case, caught somewhere between horror and truth, the scholar admits, "The smell of blood and sweat forced itself through the wall and incorporated us into what was happening inside. My own pulse beat more quickly. ... [And] instantly, I understood what a personal challenge anthropological fieldwork could be. I was witnessing 'torture', and the fact that I remained standing with the others outside somehow sanctioned what happened inside ..."[12]

My point exactly, with one proviso: anthropologists don't '*somehow* sanction' FGM. Their 'white coats' legitimize it and thereby vitiate activists' campaigns. Note that the original essay places 'torture' in quotation marks, meaning to convey, IS it REALLY torture? No, not *really* ...

But FGM *IS* torture – *sans* quotation marks. And even when anesthesia works in clinics, amputations inflict lasting wounds and violate human rights.

Yet, the good news is ...

There is good news coming out of Kenya. NGOs are making headway in efforts to stop FGM among the Maasai. Despite insistence that "'Cutting girls is something our people have done for hundreds of years. No one can convince us that it is wrong',"[13] we *can* conclude on a positive note.

Here are a few promising projects. (You can find many more...)
Cricket Without Boundaries (CWB), a UK charity founded in 2005, in cooperation with the Maasai Cricket Warriors and Esther

Njenga of 28 Too Many use the game "as a vehicle to work with local communities, empower young people and deliver important health and anti-FGM education,"[14] as they did in February 2015, coaching the sport for a week in Laikipia. Ed Williams, CWB founder, explains, "CWB has been built on our passionate belief in the power of cricket as a tool for social development. Over the last 10 years we … raise[d] awareness of HIV/AIDS, [brought] communities together, empower[ed] women and rehabilitate[d] child soldiers. The fight against FGM is a hugely important cause and a natural extension of our work."[15]

In "Good news: How FGM practices are changing among the Maasai," Chelsea White describes another project. Dr. Kakenya Ntaiya started a school where attendance is conditional on two things: "No girl will be mutilated" nor will any be married off before graduation. "Thanks to education campaigns and alternative practices FGM rates have declined… . The Maasai of Esiteti in southern Kenya have decided to give up … 'cutting', [exchanging it for] a new alternative [ceremony in which] girls between the ages of 9-12 [receive] traditional beads and clothes to mark their rite of passage into womanhood." Dancing, singing inherited songs, and learning their community's prescriptions for "women's role" appear on the two-week curriculum. When more conservative tribes also slaughter livestock, initiates may be advised "to drink the raw blood," some of which "is also sprinkled on their head to identify those who have undergone the custom." A typical reaction to the innovation is expressed by one young girl who said, "'We [really] enjoy the new ceremony because it doesn't interfere with our health and education … [nor is it] brutal like the cut'."[16]

In the same vein, the Pastoralist Child Foundation offers an alternative rite of passage for Samburu girls – cousins to the Maasai – in Kenya. The aim is "to help them voice their opposition to ancient, harmful practises," especially FGM and child marriage to which it is often linked. August 9-13, 2015, witnessed an "Alternative Rite of Passage Summer Camp" for fifty girls aged 13-17. Empowering them "to say 'NO!'" "educational workshops" that eschew the blade were "followed by ceremonies with songs, dance, poetry, drama, and ... gifts."[17]

The Pastoralist Child Foundation, Inc., founded by "a group of concerned, educated, young adult pastoralists from the Samburu and Maasai communities in Kenya, and a Canadian/American woman who visited a Samburu village while on safari in 2012," is a registered community-based organization (CBO) in Kenya with tax exempt status as a 501 (c) 3 in the USA as well. "The organization's formation is a result of caring individuals, male and female, who want to see the end of harmful cultural practices such as female genital mutilation (FGM) and forced marriages of young girls. We all agree that safe alternative rites of passage (much more fun for the girls!!) and sponsoring girls' education at the primary and secondary school levels is the way to go."[18] Sayydah Garrett is founder and president.

Preference for this approach is further confirmed by Sharon Rainey. Responding to Mona Eltahawy's superb opinion piece in *The New York Times*,[19] Rainey introduces Amref Health Africa, an African-led NGO. Also promoting "alternative rites of passage," the initiative was founded by one Maasai girl who had been spared, Nice Nailantei Leng'ete. At twenty-three, she approached tribal elders, explaining the harm of FGM. With their support, she developed a ceremony – "all the celebration and pageantry without the cut" that embraces a "three-day workshop on sexual and reproductive rights and emphasizes the importance of girls staying in school – another disastrous fallout from cutting, as girls drop out ... to be married once they're cut. So far, thousands of African girls have escaped ..."[20]

In sum, if proponents' "vehemence shows us just how entrenched this practice is,"[21] Maasai activists like Nice, Sayydah, Dr. Kakenya Ntaiya, and not least of all, Valentine and Kiminta represent a future whose trajectory aims inexorably toward renewed bodily integrity – also for girls born Maasai.

Notes

1 Edwin Nyarangi. "19-year-old woman fined Sh200,000 after undergoing FGM." *Star news* http://www.the-star.co.ke/news/19-year-old-woman-fined-sh200000-after-undergoing-fgm Retrieved 13 December 2014.

2 Ibid.

3 Aims of the AWE association website include "to empower African women; to support upcoming and existing entrepreneurs; to positively reflect the image of an African wom[a]n…" http://aweawards.africanwomenineurope.eu/?page_id=51 Retrieved 14 July 2015.

4 The 'circumcision' ceremony is called "emorata" in Maa.

5 For a fuller account of the movement against FGM in Germany see Tobe Levin's preface and introduction in Levin, Tobe and Augustine H. Asaah, eds. *Empathy and Rage. Female Genital Mutilation in African Literature.* Banbury, Oxfordshire: Ayebia Publishers, 2009; "Preface," xiv-xvii; Introduction: "Assaults on Female Genitalia: Activists, Authors and the Arts" (1-14). For an essay on the four 'foremothers' of the German anti-FGM movement – Dr. Herta Haas, Fran Hosken, Hanny Lightfoot-Klein, and Tobe Levin – see Marion A. Hulverscheidt, "Health Right or Human Rite? Changing tides in the international discussion of female genital mutilation, 1970-2010." *Assembling Health Rights in Global Context. Genealogies and Anthropologies.* Eds. Alex Mold and David Reubi. NY: Routledge, 2013. 94-108.

6 Imonikebe's painting was part of a travelling exhibition of artwork against FGM, "Through the Eyes of Nigerian Artists," that was shown in 70 venues in Germany, Switzerland and Italy between 4 February 2000 and 26 February 2006. It then flew to the USA where viewers could visit it in eight universities including Brandeis, Harvard and Cornell. See http://vc.bridgew.edu/bsu_art_shows/49/ Retrieved 16 July 2015.

7 Robert Kiplagat. "Traditionalist. Female Genital Mutilation is 'holy'." *Standard Digital* online. 19 July 2014.
http://www.standardmedia.co.ke/m/story.php?id=2000128533&pageNo=1 Retrieved 13 July 2015.

8 bid.

9 "The Crime of Female Genital Mutilation." Reprinted from *Women and Revolution* No. 41, Summer/Autumn 1992. http://www.icl-fi.org/english/womendrev/oldsite/FGM.HTM Retrieved 13 July 2015.

10 The paragraph is based on a passage in Tobe Levin. "'Highly valued by both sexes': Activists, Anthr/apologists and FGM." Rev. of Hernlund, Ylva and Bettina Shell-Duncan, eds. *Transcultural Bodies. Female Genital Cutting in Global Context.* New Brunswick: Rutgers UP, 2007. In *Journal on Female Genital Mutilation and Other Harmful Traditional Practices.* Scientific Organ of

125

IAC. IAC 25th Anniversary Commemorative Issue. Vol. 3, No. 1, 2010 (including Vol. 2 No. 2). 52-61. Critiqued is Aud Talle, "Female Circumcision in Africa and Beyond. The Anthropology of a Difficult Issue." In Hernlund & Shell-Duncan. See   http://www.accmuk.com/fgm_factsheet_1.pdf and the original, slightly longer version at   http://www.ddv-verlag.de/issn_1570_0038_FE%2009_2010.pdf

11 Ibid.

12 Ibid.

13 As Siddharth Chatterjee reminds us, quoting Nashiru, a Maasai exciser in Kenya. In Siddharth Chatterjee. "Female Genital Mutilation in Kenya. When Will It End?" *The Huffington Post* online. 20 September 2014.

http://www.huffingtonpost.com/siddharth-chatterjee/female-genital-mutilation_6_b_5851806.html Retrieved 22 September 2014.

14 "Batting FGM out of Kenya."

http://28toomany.org/news/batting-fgm-out-kenya/#sthash.C6OYaadx.dpuf

http://28toomany.org/news/batting-fgm-out-kenya/ Retrieved 9 July 2015.

15 Ibid.

16 Chelsea White. "Good news: How FGM practices are changing among the Maasai."

https://www.globalcitizen.org/en/content/good-news-how-fgm-practices-are-changing-among-the/ Retrieved 9 July 2015.

17 http://pastoralist-child-foundation.org/about-us/ Retrieved 13 July 2015.

18 Ibid.

19 Mona Eltahawy. "Fighting Female Genital Mutilation." *New York Times* online. 16 November 2014

http://www.nytimes.com/2014/11/17/opinion/fighting-female-genital-mutilation.html?emc=edit_ty_20141117&nl=opinion&nlid=44488146&_r=1 Retrieved 14 July 2015.

20 Ibid.

21 Qtd. by Chatterjee (note 13).

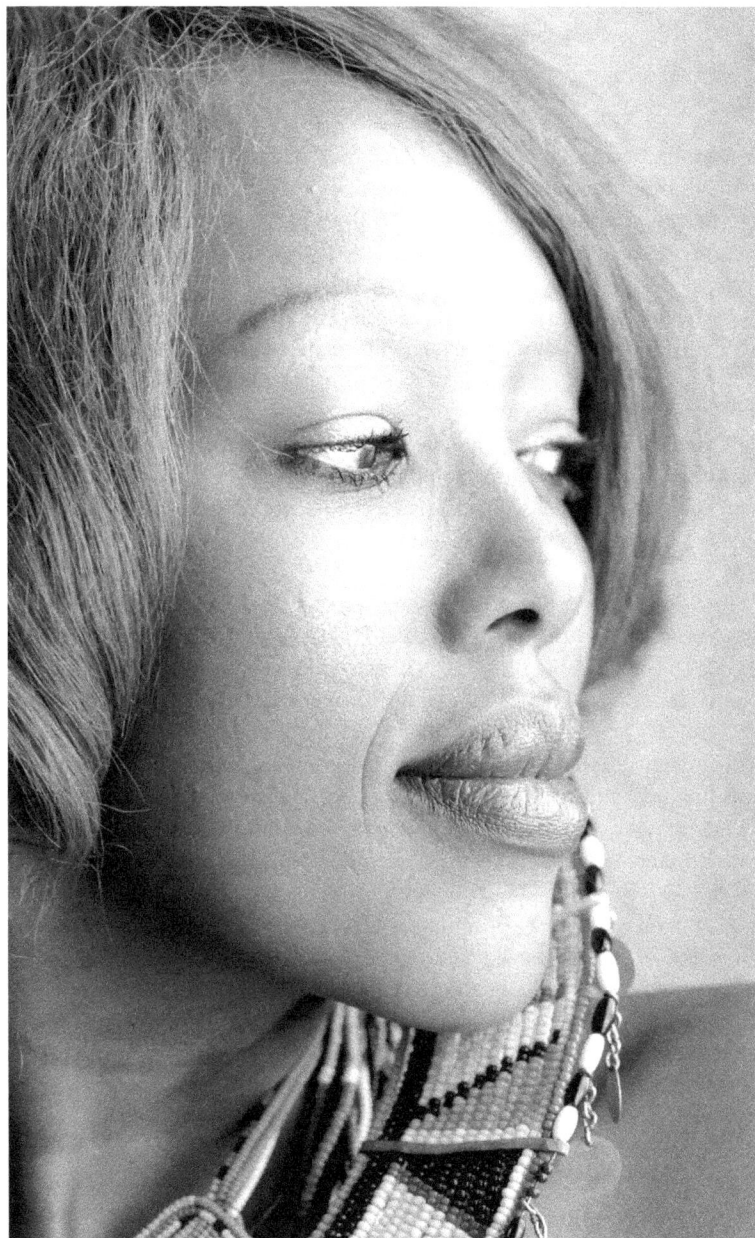

AFTERWORD

Maria Kiminta

Born on December 25, 1978, in Narok, Kenya, I am the daughter of Maasai parents, the fifth child of my father, a cow herder, and my mother who worked in community development. Both parents had a great sense of humor.

Fortunate to attend university in Nairobi, I pursued my interest in advancing women's human rights in various villages but then traded my dream of advocating human betterment for a more pragmatic career in sales. My first job in a women's clothing store led to engagement to the owner's son followed by marriage and moving to Germany. Europe has enabled me to return to my passion for helping women discover the irrelevance and detriment to health of the ritual passage so many of us had been through. I aim to promote confidence and education among Maasai girls.

In Germany, I appeared at several modest meetings including one at the Seventh Day Adventist Church in Bad Segeberg with the theme STOP FGM. This led to a big break in 2012 when I rescued one girl out of the 134 forced to face the knife back in my Maasai community. That was the start.

The mantra, education, on which my personal growth is based, holds out the most hope for girls suffering poor health, and especially sexual ill-health, associated with 'circumcision' including HIV, easily spread by practitioners failing to abide by basic antiseptic measures.

I can't tell whether the horrendous dénouement of my mutilation resulted from the operator's negligent hygiene, but that I suffered greatly had a huge effect on the woman and campaigner I have become, someone keen to ensure girls know about their right to be free from the risk of FGM and enabled to grow up free from violence and fear.

What happened to me? When giving birth I was afforded the confidence to confide in my empathetic gynecologist, Dr. rer. nat. Ralph Rathmann concerning the genital torture I had undergone, telling him about the severe pain and prolonged healing period full of problems like excessive bleeding I was unable to stop and difficulty in urination and defecation due to hardened stool made almost impossible to pass by swelling of surrounding tissue. I remember the noxious odor as well coming from my wounded, infected vagina. Still very young at the time, I recall all this clearly. What I never found out was what kind of infection, four weeks after the cutting, I still had …

For remember, 'surgical' tools are used without sterilization, and the same blade is at times applied to twenty girls or more. In my case, we were three cut with the same razor held in hands without gloves. Every day I'm grateful to be neither HIV-positive nor dead.

But a *BIG* scar remains on my vagina and my mind. Trauma memory, I call it. And I ask myself again and again, who should have helped me, protected me? Who could have treated my nerve pain, or the abscess or ulcers that developed? And what about the back pain, unstoppable urine and urinary tract infections with their own flaying scorch?

Unlike my girlfriends, my sexual life is not very active probably because my clitoris has been cut off and my sensitive vaginal tissue scarred. Yes, I have sexual feeling but I take longer to reach fulfilment and only after fighting hard to disassociate the act from the brutality of FGM done to me as a young girl.

And the cutting goes on. In labor, I wanted a caesarean section, fearing inability to stand more vaginal pain and unwilling to lose my child to FGM-related complications. I anticipated the anxiety, depression, and stress I knew would come with anything related to the genitals, and feared I might go crazy if allowed to face the same intensity of pain I had gone through with FGM. And let's not forget defloration, another hell.

Although a patient partner has enabled me to attain a level of comfort in my sex life, I now know that FGM damages health not only right away, in the young girls that are its victims, but in the long term in grown-up women as well.

I dedicate this book to all supporters of children's rights and to the young girls who, after reading my story, will know that rituals like FGM don't make life complete; on the contrary. Now enabled to say no, youth will face life not revering a culture of harm but respecting education for good.

NO to FGM.

Defining Womanhood as Pain … on FGM

Airyn Lentija-Sloan

Gone were her smiles while there she lay,
Hearing the cries of another girl …
Dread in her nerves and muscles taut as
Tradition inflamed her world.

On either side, with all their strength, old women
held on, preventing escape
and forced her to bear the blight of blades.
What unspeakable pain at such a young age!

Struggling just to remain alive
She hurled her grief at an unhearing pride.
Resistance reached a frenzied pitch.
Then they began to stitch.

One with the earth, her face in tears
Her body invaded by so many fears
She wanted to ask why she suffered like this
But slowly fell blank and lost consciousness.

NOTES ON CONTRIBUTORS

Noel Siqi Duan received her master's degree in women's studies from the University of Oxford in 2014. A Columbia University graduate class of 2013, she studied sociocultural anthropology and art history, working extensively with ethnography on the Maasai. Her general interests are in gendered bodies, postcolonial activism, sweatshop labor, fashion history, sustainability and consum-erism, feminist art, technology, and women's media. She has written for *Teen Vogue, ELLE, Oxford Times, xoJane, Wonderland,* and other cultural publications. She currently resides in Brooklyn, New York, and San Francisco, California.

Equality Now is a registered charity that protects and promotes "the human rights of women and girls around the world. Working with grass-roots women's and human rights organizations and individual activists since 1992, Equality Now documents violence and discrimination against women and mobilizes international action to support efforts to stop these abuses." http://www.equalitynow.org/about-us

IRIN News is a non-profit agency that until 1 January 2015 had been associated with the UN but has since become independent. Its acronym stands for Integrated Regional Information Networks, and it describes it-self as "a news agency focusing on humanitarian stories in regions that are often forgotten, under-reported, misunderstood or ignored." It was founded in Kenya. http://newirin.irinnews.org/landing/

Maria Kiminta, a courageous, outspoken Maasai lives in northern Ger-many and is the proud mother of a newborn girl …

Airyn Lentija-Sloan, born in the Philippines, is a poet, most of whose works are published in *Human Rights and Culture*, an e-publication of the Asian Human Rights Commission. "Defining Womanhood as Pain: On FGM" first appeared in *Feminist Europa. Review of Books.* Special Issue on FGM (2009/2010). Airyn blogs at http://airynspoetry.blogspot.com

Tobe Levin von Gleichen holds a Ph.D. in comparative literature from Cornell University, is a professor emerita (University of Maryland UC Europe), a Visiting Research Fellow in International Gender Studies at Lady Margaret Hall, University of Oxford and an Associate, the Hutchins Center for Af-rican and African-American Research, Harvard University. An activist against FGM since 1977, she co-founded FORWARD-Germany in 1998 and in

2009 launched UnCUT/VOICES Press focusing on FGM where she serves as author, editor, translator, and publisher.

Audrey Matere, with an undergraduate major in educational communication and technology, is an expert in e-education and Coordinator in the Faculty of Education and Human Resource Development at Kisii University (Eldoret Campus), Kenya.

Valentine Nkoyo completed her MBA at Nottingham Trent University. A Business Management graduate from York St. John University, she is a human rights advocate, public speaker, promoter of education and FGM activist. Her passion to support others, mainly girls and women, derives from her own experiences of FGM when aged 11 and from fighting to escape poverty and discrimination while growing up. She focuses on eradicating FGM, empowering girls and women through education, and acting to enhance health. Director of the Mojatu Foundation, a community organization that works closely with African and Caribbean communities in media, health and education to stop FGM, she is also editor of Mojatu publications. Valentine has won several awards including International Student of the Year for Yorkshire and the Humber Region from the British Council for contribution to cultural diversity awareness of UK institutions and community support. See https://vimeo.com/10067804

Peter Gutwa Oino is Programme Officer at Ex-Street Children Organization and a part-time lecturer in the Faculty of Arts and Social Sciences at Kisii University (Eldoret Campus), Department of Social Sciences, P.O. Box, 6434-30100, Eldoret, Kenya. With Geofrey Towett, he is co-author of "The Dilemma in Sustainability of Community-Based Projects in Kenya" that appeared in *Global Journal of Advanced Research*, Vol. 2 No. 4. See <http://www.gjar.org/publishpaper/vol2issue4/d177r18.pdf>

Britta Radike, freelance photographer in Essen, concentrates on corporate PR, people photography and portraits. A student of geography, ethnology and psychology at Humboldt University and the Free University of Berlin, she received a DAAD (German Academic Exchange Service) fellowship to the University of Applied Sciences and Art in Dortmund, Germany. Her thesis, a book about ethnic Somali refugees from Ogaden in the Horn of Africa, led to "A Place to Call Home. Images and Interviews with Refugees from Ogaden" (with Tobe Levin) in *Transition. An International Review*. An official publication of Harvard University. (Vol. 110, 2008. 78-11). In 2007, Radike participated in the TPW Masterclass with Stanley Greene and Kadir von Lohuizen in Italy. In addition, a grant from the "VG

Bildkunst" (German cultural department of the copyright collective for pictures and art) facilitated an extensive report on orphaned children in Rwanda 15 years after the genocide. In 2011 she and Sebastian Christ were nominated for a CNN Journalist Award for documenting the German mission in Afghanistan. To her credit, Radike has other photographic projects in many Middle Eastern nations, in South-East Asia, Latin America and the Caribbean as well as in Uganda, Kenya, Eritrea, Ethiopia, and Burundi. She is a member of FORWARD – Germany against FGM.

Geofrey Towett is Coordinator at the Faculty of Arts and Social Sciences at Kisii University (Eldoret Campus), Kenya, specializing in Development Studies, International Relations and Human Rights Law. His most recent article on FGM can be cited as Geofrey Towett, Peter Gutwa Oino, Gatobu Caroline, and Pauline Tarkwen, "Socio-Cultural Factors Influencing the Practice of Female Genital Cut among the Maasai Community of Kajiado Central Sub-County, Kenya," *International Journal of Innovation and Scientific Research*, vol. 13, no. 1, pp. 186–192, January 2015.

Each UnCUT/VOICES Press book supports a specific project against FGM. Sales of *Kiminta* contribute to the **Clitoris Restoration Fund** that sponsors operations by Dr. Pierre Foldes at the Institut Génésique in St. Germain-en-Laye outside Paris, France.

In the United States, your donation is tax deductible. Send a check in any amount made out to **Healthy Tomorrow** with a clear notation that you are contributing to the Clitoris Restoration Fund.

The address: **Healthy Tomorrow, 14 William St., Somerville, MA 02144 USA.**

You can also make a tax-deductible contribution in Germany by bank transfer to FORWARD –Germany with the clear notation **Clitoris Restoration Fund and your email or snail-mail address**. (For tax deduction in other European nations, please ask your income tax authority if a German Spendenquittung/ receipt will be honored.)

Make bank transfers to
FORWARD – Germany e.V.
Frankfurter Sparkasse
BLZ 500 502 01
Account # 200029398
IBAN: DE20 5005 0201 0200 0293 98
BIC SWIFT: HELADEF1822

A UK charity is in formation. For details, watch the website <www.uncutvoices.wordpress.com>.

136